OXFORD MEDICAL PUBLICATIONS

Clinical epidemiology of stroke

Clinical epidemiology of stroke

SHAH EBRAHIM

Professor of Health Care of the Elderly,
The London Hospital Medical College,
London

Oxford New York Toronto
OXFORD UNIVERSITY PRESS
1990

Oxford University Press, Walton Street, Oxford OX2 6DP
Oxford New York Toronto
Delhi Bombay Calcutta Madras Karachi
Petaling Jaya Singapore Hong Kong Tokyo
Nairobi Dar es Salaam Cape Town
Melbourne Auckland
and associated companies in
Berlin Ibadan

Oxford is a trade mark of Oxford University Press

Published in the United States
by Oxford University Press, New York

British Library Cataloguing in Publication Data
Ebrahim, Shah B. J.
The clinical epidemiology of stroke.
1. Man. Brain. Strokes
I. Title
616.81
ISBN 0-19-261749-4

Library of Congress Cataloging in Publication Data
Ebrahim, Shah.
Clinical epidemiology of stroke / Shah Ebrahim.
(Oxford medical publications)
Includes bibliographical references.
1. Cerebrovascular disease—Epidemiology. I. Title. II. Series.
[DNLM: 1. Cerebrovascular Disorders—epidemiology. WL 355 E16c]
RC388.5.E27 1990 614.5'981—dc20 90-7137
ISBN 0-19-261749-4

Typeset by Downdell Limited, Oxford
Printed in Great Britain by
Biddles Ltd, Guildford and King's Lynn

Foreword

Stroke is a tragedy. Stroke victims who have written about their experiences tell us that their illness is probably the most significant event that they have ever experienced. One described stroke as being more momentous than marriage, or having children, or the stages of one's career. Another said it was the most terrifying experience of her life. Yet cerebrovascular disease does not necessarily engender medical interest. Perhaps because stroke is so common, there is a tendency for some health professionals to consider it as a mundane condition, devoid of interest, and lacking in intellectual challenge. In the past, most research concentrated on the search for the magic bullet, the pharmacological agent which would limit cerebral damage or accelerate recovery. This quest has been generally disappointing and bright young research workers have tended to look to other areas of endeavour which might yield more fruitful results.

Consequently the approach to stroke has tended to be nihilistic. This has been recognized by patients and their families, some of whom have viewed doctors as shadowy figures, who did not offer comfort but seemed embarrassed, as if they did not know what to do. Stroke rehabilitation in particular was seen as a no-man's land in which disabled survivors were left untended to grope their way alone.

In recent years, attitudes have begun to change. Energetic and enthusiastic people from different disciplines have applied themselves vigorously to improving the care of stroke patients and their families. Shah Ebrahim is one of these. Before taking up his chair in Medicine for the Elderly at the London Hospital, Shah worked in Nottingham, where he had trained as an undergraduate. Here he developed a passion for clinical enquiry and a sense of constructive criticism. Work in the Department of Health Care of the Elderly in Nottingham provided exposure to the psychological aspects of illness and to the challenges of rehabilitation. His spell in general practice provided a broader view of medicine and his continuing commitment to Third World countries has added a global dimension.

By developing expertise in epidemiology, Shah has further equipped himself to make a very special contribution to the world of stroke care. This important book reflects his eclecticism.

There are several themes which permeate this monograph. The first is an emphasis on the importance of well designed clinical trials. Professor Ebrahim analyses the published studies, points out flaws in the design of some of them, and provides helpful interpretations of results. Secondly he questions our reliance on clinical experience: personal inconsistency and poor inter-observer agreement on basic physical signs should act as a stimulus to re-evaluate our skills in the clinical examination of our patients.

Thirdly he points to the gaps in our knowledge, providing ideas for future research and offering practical advice where the paucity of hard data make informed decision-making impossible.

We are gently introduced to the vocabulary of epidemiology and shown the great importance of this science in the development of better forms of stroke care. The descriptions of the many rating scales now available for the assessment of different aspects of stroke illness are particularly valuable. Professor Ebrahim's emphasis on numeracy and cost–benefit analysis is nicely balanced by his compassionate attitude towards disabled patients and empathy towards over-burdened relatives.

By challenging assumptions, questioning time-hallowed practices and showing the ways forward, Professor Ebrahim has produced a provocative, thoughtful and eminently sensible book. Experts in stroke will learn much from it; those who are relatively new to the field will be inspired; busy clinicians who scan the useful summaries at the end of each chapter will want to delve more deeply.

This is an important addition to the stroke literature. I am sure that you will enjoy reading it as much as I have.

Professor G.P. Mulley
Department of Medicine for the Elderly,
St James's University Hospital, Leeds

Preface

Epidemiology is a basic medical science that is fundamental to understanding diagnosis, treatment, and prognosis.

Diagnosis requires answers to a series of questions: is this patient sick or well? If sick, what are the chances of a particular disease causing the problem? What investigations will be most useful in obtaining the diagnosis? Epidemiology applied to the bedside problems of patients—clinical epidemiology—can help to provide solutions. The ability of a detail of the patient's history, or a clinical sign which could rule in or out a diagnosis can be described by using simple arithmetic. The probability that a disease is or is not present can be given a numerical value, and the extent to which investigation increases or reduces the likelihood of discovering disease can also be measured.

Deciding on the treatment to give a patient is dependent on understanding what clinical trials and other observational studies tell us. It is necessary to appreciate the extent to which a trial is relevant to one's own clinical practice, the possibilities of biases, and of low power studies, which may invalidate conclusions drawn from trials. The most effective treatments have risks, and to weigh adequately the benefits and the risks of treatment the clinician needs a more accurate scale than past experience or intuition. Quantifying benefit and risk can be done using rates, often expressed as events per 100 or 1000 patients treated. The techniques to describe these types of information belong to clinical epidemiology.

Prognosis is something that most patients and their relatives want to hear about. Prognosis for survival, for functional recovery, or chances of complications are all aspects of measuring the consequences of disease. The concepts underlying measurement of the impact of disease on patients can now be broadly classified, and a more complete appraisal given. This in turn should provide the spur to look for ways of improving prognosis, of concentrating on areas that have been neglected, yet may hold the key to improving our patients' quality of life.

In addition to underpinning these fundamental principles of medical practice—diagnosis, treatment, and prognosis—epidemiology provides ways of examining causality. The role of the hospital clinician in leading preventive care for individual patients is limited largely to secondary prevention, i.e. stopping the problem recurring (or getting worse) after it has become established. However, primary care physicians have a clear role in primary prevention, which in the case of stroke means modification of risk factors. Epidemiology gives an indication of which risk factors merit intervention because of their large attributable risks.

The best way to learn about a disease is to gain considerable clinical experience from an acknowledged expert of the disease. Clinical experience is a slow and often very biased way of learning about a disease—the patients seen by the specialist are usually very dissimilar to those seen by more ordinary doctors.

Information gained by the experiential method is difficult to collect, sort, make sense of, and even more difficult to recollect when needed. It may seem paradoxical that the techniques of epidemiology—a population science—should be applicable to the problems of individual patients. To a large extent this is because the best estimates we have of what will happen to an individual undergoing diagnosis or treatment is derived not from clinical experience, but from the experience of a large number of similar patients. Until we have the ability to make predictions for individuals derived from their innate characteristics, the experience of groups of patients will be highly relevant to clinical practice.

Unfortunately, the skills that make clinical medicine appealing do not seem to be the same as those that make arithmetic easy. I have been struck by the major difficulties bright medical students have found in carrying out division and multiplication, to arrive at measures such as sensitivity and specificity of a test. Throughout this book examples have been worked out with all the necessary stages included to help the innumerate see the way. The numbers are not essential to understanding the messages of this book, and those of you who are put off by the sight of equations can simply skip them. A second problem is the use of epidemiological jargon. I make no apologies for using accepted epidemiological words that deserve to be part of a clinician's working vocabulary more than incomprehensible terms used by clinicians such as pseudo-pseudo-hyperparathyroidism!

Stroke is one of the most common diagnoses made by physicians, yet the disease does not have much appeal. Patients with signs and symptoms suggestive of stroke require careful assessment to avoid diagnostic error. The value of investigation, in particular neuroradiology, is debatable. Treatments exist, but a sense of therapeutic nihilism prevails. The prognosis of stroke looks gloomy viewed from medical wards where patients wait for transfer to some other place. This book aims to examine these and other questions of diagnosis, treatment, and prognosis of stroke using epidemiological methods. Answers to questions are always in short supply, and if the reader finds a lack of dogmatic statement and a surfeit of data and discussion, then the book may have achieved another goal—that of encouraging sceptical thought.

This book is written by a clinician who is also trained in epidemiology, and is intended for clinicians who treat patients with stroke, for epidemiologists who want to apply epidemiology to clinical problems, for therapists who wish to develop their understanding of the application of scientific method to rehabilitation practice, and for medical students who may wish to accelerate and complement the process of acquiring clinical experience about stroke.

London S.B.J.E.
January 1990

To

Maurice Backett and Tom Arie who showed me the way

and

Julia, who kept me on it.

Contents

Part I

Diagnosis

1 Risk and risk factors

What caused the stroke?

In common with most chronic diseases, strokes do not have single causes, but seem to be multifactorial in their causation. However, even in infectious diseases that have a single cause, such as mycobacterium tuberculosis, the risk of being infected, and then of developing tuberculosis, is dependent on a chain of causal factors, some very closely related to the pathogenetic process (e.g. inhaling bacilli from a close relative), whereas others are much further back in the causal chain (e.g. poor childhood nutrition). Epidemiologists are frequently concerned with discovering characteristics of people and populations that increase or decrease their chances (or risk) of suffering diseases. The mechanisms by which disease occurs in those at increased risk is often suggested by epidemiological enquiry, but working out the final pathological pathways is a goal for laboratory scientists.

The question of causation can be answered at several different levels: what are the precipitants that cause a person to have a stroke on a particular day; what pathological processes are going on in the cardiovascular system that impair the cerebral circulation; what predisposes people to have strokes? These questions are concerned with why strokes occur, but at different points along a chain of causality which starts with DNA and genes, goes on to the modification of genetic expression by environmental factors, to produce a person with more or less predisposition to cerebrovascular diseases. The person is then influenced by a series of environmental exposures, some of which can be controlled by individuals (e.g. cigarette smoking, diet, inactivity) and some of which cannot (e.g. climate, water, air quality). These fundamental and predisposing causes lead to the occurrence of strokes through pathogenetic mechanisms involving blood vessels, blood components, blood pressure, and flow dynamics.

The purpose of studying causes more fundamental than the pathological process is that such causes lend themselves to attempts at disease prevention. Linking risk of diarrhoeal diseases with water quality can lead to disease control without any need to understand that a bacterium is responsible for the pathological process. The current HIV epidemic is a good example of how knowledge of risk factors can lead to preventive activity before any clear understanding of the mechanism by which the virus affects the immune system. Understanding mechanisms may be rewarded by discovering new treatments for a disease, thus enquiry into aetiology and pathogenesis are complementary.

Criteria to establish causality

Causality is difficult to ascertain accurately, but Koch's postulates define standard criteria that should be met before a claim of causality can be accepted. These postulates are essentially to do with specificity of a relationship between an organism and a disease. The organism must be found with the disease and not with any other disease, and the isolated organism must be capable of causing the disease in susceptible subjects. Koch's postulates enabled the single necessary cause of an infectious disease to be established, but in chronic diseases single necessary causes have been comparatively rare. Perhaps exposure to tobacco and lung cancer comes closest to the infectious disease model of a single cause, but even so many who do smoke will not develop lung cancer and therefore predisposing and protective factors presumably operate to determine its occurrence.

The major problem which has beset stroke epidemiology from the outset, is that the pathological damage that leads to a stroke is not a single process but may be due to thrombosis of arteries, platelet emboli from the carotid arteries, fibrin emboli from the atrium, increased viscosity of blood, or rupture of microaneurysms of intracerebral arteries. Yet the clinical presentation of stroke is remarkably similar whatever the pathogenesis, and until recently accurate discrimination between the major mechanisms, thrombosis and haemorrhage, has not been possible. This has led to much of our understanding of causation being weakened because environmental and personal factors that increase risk (risk factors) have been measured as if strokes were a single disease. The first prerequisite to establish causality is to ensure that the disease of interest is as homogeneous an entity as is possible given current knowledge about disease mechanisms. Other sub-categories of the major mechanisms of haemorrhage and infarction (e.g. haemorrhagic infarction, embolic infarction) may be less relevant in epidemiological enquiry as they simply represent the location or severity of the disease, rather than any fundamental difference in aetiology.

The other criteria of aetiological causality were originally framed by Hill (1965) and comprise:

(1) strength of association of a risk factor with the disease;
(2) experiment (changing the risk factor leads to changes in disease occurrence);
(3) dose-response effect (more of a risk factor leads to more disease);
(4) time sequence (a risk factor must exert its effect before disease appears);
(5) consistency (similar associations in other places and times among different people);
(6) biological plausibility, coherence with other information;
(7) specificity of association (a risk factor is only associated with a particular disease);
(8) analogy with other examples of cause and effect.

The first five of these criteria are the most powerful in establishing causality because the others are bound by existing knowledge, and specificity of a relationship may not be a helpful criterion as smoking, for example, is a causal factor of several different diseases.

Risk

The term 'risk' is widely used to indicate the level of disease occurrence—incidence or prevalence, depending on the disease. For diseases with an acute onset, such as myocardial infarction and stroke, risk is usually equated with incidence—the number of new cases of disease arising over a defined time period among a defined population at risk of the disease.

Epidemiology, like any science, draws inferences from empirical observations most of which require comparisons. A simple comparison of the *number* of cases of stroke occurring in two places, or at two times, would clearly be subject to the obvious defect that one place may have a greater population and therefore more cases. This basic concept of *a population at risk* is necessary for valid comparisons to be made. To make appropriate comparisons it is necessary to compare like with like and the epidemiological tool for this purpose is the *rate*. Incidence rates are proportions that are comprised of a numerator (the number of new cases in a period of time) and a denominator which is the number of people at risk of the disease over the same time.

When incidence rates are measured over several years, the population at risk will change as time passes. The most obvious change will be ageing, but some people will leave the area, others will move in, some will die, some will have a stroke and pass from the denominator to the numerator. Deciding on the denominator can be done by assuming that the population resident in the area at the mid-point of the study is a good enough approximation to the population at risk over the whole period. For rare diseases this usually is good enough because the numerator is always tiny compared with the denominator and small changes in the denominator will have little impact on the incidence rate. For more common diseases, like stroke and ischaemic heart disease, it is necessary to measure the population at risk in terms of *person-years at risk*. A person followed for 10 years contributes 10 person-years of risk to the denominator, 10 people followed for one year also contribute 10 person-years of risk.

Individual risk

The crude incidence of stroke in several collaborating general practices in Oxford was 1.64 per 1000 person-years at risk, but varied dramatically with age, more than doubling for every decade from the age of 55 (Oxford Community Stroke Project 1983; Bamford *et al.* 1988). Incidence rates give the best approximation available for an individual's chances of having a stroke in the absence of any other information about the individual. It is curious that the estimates derived from large numbers of people give the best information we have about individuals, but this has long been known by insurance companies which base their premiums (their estimates of risk of dying) on accumulated information about disease incidence at different ages (the major factor), for each sex, in different occupations, and for different body builds, blood pressures, and smoking behaviour.

Consequently, for a woman in Oxford aged 60 years, the risk of having a stroke if nothing else is known about her (e.g. blood pressure, smoking history, presence of heart disease, diabetes, etc.) is 2.95 per 1000 person-years at risk, which is equivalent to an annual risk of 0.00295 for a single woman-year at risk or less than a third of 1 per cent a year. At 70 years, the same women will have an annual risk of stroke of 0.00689. This is still a small risk, less than 1 per cent, but is a big increase compared with 10 years earlier; a greater than two-fold increase.

Of course, this assumes that the risk of stroke experienced by 70-year-olds now will be the same in 10 years time, that is, that the magnitude of the cross-sectional observation that stroke incidence increases with age will apply to subsequent cohorts of younger people as they age. Mortality rates for stroke can be used as a proxy for incidence rates (which are not routinely available over long time periods) to examine whether this assumption is reasonable. The striking finding is that mortality rates from stroke have shown a consistent decline over many years, and this does not appear to be a cohort phenomenon (i.e. it is not due to a high risk group of people moving through from birth to death, to be replaced by lower risk people). Each age band, including the very old have enjoyed lower death rates from stroke (Whisnant 1984). This secular, or period, effect suggests that some factor which has a uniform impact on the occurrence of stroke at all ages has changed for the better over the last 40 years.

Risk ratio and odds ratio

Comparisons between people with different characteristics requires the incidence rate in one group to be compared with the incidence rate in the other. Taking the change in risk of a stroke for the Oxford woman at age 60 and age 70, the risk ratio (which may be called a rate ratio or a relative risk) is simply the ratio of the incidence at 70 to the incidence at 60 years: $0.00689/0.00292 = 2.36$. The risk ratio disguises the fairly low incidence rates which can lead to inappropriate alarm if a person considers that simply by living another 10 years they have a 236 per cent increased risk of having a stroke! Risk ratios are extremely useful when looking for potential causes of stroke because they are good measures of the strength of association between a factor and disease.

They are of limited use in clinical practice when the baseline risk is much more relevant to the patient and doctor. The woman of 70 asking about her increased chances of having a stroke should not be told that her risk is now over 200 per cent of what it was 10 years earlier, but that her risk has increased by $0.00689 - 0.00292 = 0.00397$ per year, or rather less than one-half per cent a year. As most people do not think in probabilities it is usual to express a probability of 0.00397 as the number of events that would occur to a population of 100 or 1000 people. In this case, among a group of 1000 women aged 70, around four would be expected to have a stroke over the year. The absolute difference in the two rates is of vital importance in the clinical assessment of risk and gives a baseline perspective that the relative differences cannot.

Measuring risk ratios

Case control studies are often used for aetiological investigation but do not give direct measures of disease incidence because they are cross-sectional and the time frame is frozen at a point in time. The principle of a case control study is that a comparison of the frequency of a putative risk factor among cases with the disease and controls is made. The comparison may be made in two ways: the rate ratio and the odds ratio. Table 1.1 illustrates the calcu-

Table 1.1 The relationship between the rate ratio and the odds ratio

Risk factor	*Disease occurrence*		
	Present	*Absent*	
Present	a	b	$a+b$
Absent	c	d	$c+d$

Risk of disease if risk factor present: $a/(a+b)$

Rate ratio: $\dfrac{a/(a+b)}{c/(c+d)}$

Risk of disease if risk factor absent: $c/(c+d)$

If the disease is rare, i.e. a and c are small compared with b and d:

$$a/(a+b) = a/b \text{ and } c/(c+d) = c/d.$$

and the rate ratio simplifies to:

$$(a/b)/(c/d) = a \times d/b \times c = \text{the odds ratio.}$$

lations. For rare diseases, the odds ratio is a good estimate of the true risk (or rate) ratio.

In a longitudinal study where subjects are classified according to the presence or absence of risk factor(s) and the occurrence of strokes are then counted as time passes, the true rate ratios can be calculated. In a case-control study where the starting point is a group of patients who have suffered a stroke and a control group that do not have a stroke, the presence or absence of risk factors is then measured *after* the event of the stroke. The true rate of stroke in each risk factor group cannot be measured using a case control study because the proportions of stroke patients to controls have been fixed by the design (e.g. one stroke matched to one control). The odds ratio can, however, be used as a convenient proxy for the rate ratio, provided that the disease in question is relatively uncommon. The more common the disease, the less good is the odds ratio as an approximation of the true rate ratio.

For example, a case control study of the impact of smoking on stroke has been reported (Bonita *et al.* 1986) which demonstrated a three-fold increased risk of stroke among smokers compared with current non-smokers. By contrast, information from the placebo group of a large longitudinal trial of effects of antihypertensive drugs has also been used to estimate the association between smoking and stroke (MRC Working Party 1988). These data are shown in Table 1.2. The odds-ratio tends to *overestimate* the true rate ratio, but provided the disease frequency is less than about 1 per cent, then this effect is not marked.

Hypertension and smoking seem to have stronger effects when studied in a cross-sectional survey than in a longitudinal design. This is not too surprising because biases can affect cross-sectional studies more frequently than longitudinal ones. It is possible that recall bias has led to cases more often giving (or being asked more thoroughly) a history of smoking. Cross-sectional surveys can only study survivors, and it is possible that smoking and hypertension are linked with survival as well as incidence. It is clear that both smoking and hypertension are consistently related to risk of stroke regardless of the method of study.

Combining risk factors

An advantage of the rate ratio (and odds ratio) compared with absolute differences in risk is that the combined effects of two or

Table 1.2 Smoking and risk of stroke: case control vs. longitudinal estimates of risk (data taken from Bonita *et al.* 1986 and MRC Working Party 1985). Note that denominators for the MRC longitudinal study are approximate, and that the odds ratio estimates are unadjusted and hence do not equal figures reported in the studies

	Case control study		Longitudinal study	
	Stroke		Stroke	
Smoking	*Yes*	*No*	*Yes*	*No*
Yes	66	424	48	2420
No	66	1162	60	5970
Odds ratio:	$\frac{66 \times 1162}{66 \times 424} = 2.74$		$\frac{48 \times 5970}{60 \times 2420} = 1.97$	
Rate ratio:	Not applicable		$\frac{48/2468}{60/6030} = 1.95$	

more risk factors can be taken into account to give an estimate of the risk of disease. Relative risks usually combine in a multiplicative way. For example, smoking increases the risk of stroke by about two to three times, and hypertension increases risk by about four to five times. The combined effects of both smoking and hypertension might be estimated to be between 8 and 15 (i.e. 2×4 and 3×5) fold increased risk, assuming that the risks multiplied. The increased risk among hypertensive smokers observed in one case-control study was almost 20-fold (Bonita *et al.* 1986) implying that the effects of these two risk factors are multiplicative. However, another longitudinal study found only a six-fold increased risk among male hypertensive smokers (Salonen *et al.* 1982), which suggests an additive relationship between these risk factors.

A multiplicative relationship between these risk factors implies that each risk factor is operating via a different pathogenetic mechanism. Smoking may be having its effects through blood viscosity or platelet function, whereas blood pressure may be causing vessel wall damage. Additive relationships between risk factors suggest that their effects are mediated through the same pathogenic mechanisms.

A genetic predisposition to stroke

Family history

Do strokes run in the family? Strokes are common and share risk factors with the major cause of death in Western countries, ischaemic heart disease, and therein lies the problem of trying to estimate whether a family history of stroke indicates a predisposition or chance. Family studies are a weak method of assessing genetic predisposition because families share more than genetic material (Gurling 1984). A Swedish study of a cohort of men born in 1913 examined the question of the effect of a family history, looking at the effect of a maternal or paternal history of stroke. A maternal history of stroke increased risk of stroke by three-fold, after allowing for the effects of blood pressure, plasma fibrinogen, and obesity (Welin *et al.* 1987). However, in this study other accepted risk factors for stroke did not appear to be important, suggesting that the sample may be atypical.

Among relatively affluent Americans aged between 50 and 79, recruited into a longitudinal study, 25 per cent of the men and 35 per cent of the women gave a family history of stroke in a first-degree relative. In women this history was associated with a 2.3-fold increased risk of stroke over the following 12 years, and in men with a 3.3-fold increased risk of myocardial infarction but no effect on stroke (Khaw *et al.* 1986). The effects of age, cholesterol, blood pressure, smoking, and diabetes were all controlled.

Although family history of stroke is associated with an increase of systolic blood pressure of up to 10 mmHg (Sigurdsson *et al.* 1983; Miall *et al.* 1967), the association of family history with stroke is independent of its effect on blood pressure and other risk factors. A substantial familial effect exists, but it is not clear whether the family effect operates through other unknown risk factors for stroke which were not allowed for in these studies or through a genetic component of increased susceptibility to stroke. The differential effects between men and women are difficult to explain, but it may be that the familial risk in men operates at an earlier age when the chances of having a myocardial infarction are higher than having a stroke. Alternatively, female sex hormones may be relatively more cardio-protective than stroke protective.

Twin studies

Studies of the occurrence of disease among identical and dissimilar twins provide the strongest evidence of genetic predisposition. Case reports of association of a stroke between identical twins are of limited value in assessing the true genetic component of increased risk of stroke, partly because strokes are common and may occur in both twins by chance, and partly because of the bias produced by selecting twins for study because one of them has the disease of interest. The only sound methodology for studying common diseases amongst twins is to use twin registers and to examine the concordance of stroke in identical (monozygotic) and non-identical (dizygotic) twins. This avoids selection bias and allowance can be made for the expected chance association. Only one such twin study has been reported using data from the Swedish Twin Registry (De Faire *et al.* 1975). Ischaemic heart disease deaths were twice as likely among monozygotic (MZ) as dizygotic (DZ) male twins with a similar but less pronounced pattern in female twins. The concordance rates for stroke deaths were similar among both MZ and DZ twins for both male and female twins. However, stroke deaths were up to 20 times as common as expected in both types of twins, which implies that a shared family environment is an extremely strong risk factor for stroke.

It is unlikely that genetic factors have a role in risk of stroke, except through their association with ischaemic heart disease. The influence of the intra-uterine environment or early family life on subsequent risk of stroke is supported by a study that demonstrated a strong association between geographical variation in maternal mortality in 1911–14 and the stroke death rates among the cohort born at that time (Barker and Osmond 1987). The association might be mediated through risk of high blood pressure which is related to low birth weight (Gennser *et al.* 1988), and tends to show a familial relationship (Havlik *et al.* 1979; Miall and Oldham 1963). A twin study has demonstrated that multi-infarct dementia affecting both twin-pairs is associated with a much higher chance of a parental history of stroke (Jarvik and Matsuyama 1983). It is therefore possible that a genetic effect is operating to make strokes more likely but not sufficiently severe to cause death.

Further twin studies might examine the concordance in strokes between twins brought up together and apart, examining in addition the time of separation. This sort of analysis is becoming feasible as cohorts of twins separated during World War II get older and suffer strokes. This will help distinguish whether very early environments or intrauterine influences are affecting subsequent stroke risk.

Homocystinuria

This is an autosomal recessively inherited inborn error of metabolism which causes skeletal defects (similar to Marfan's syndrome), lens dislocation, and mental retardation. It also causes a tendency to both venous and thrombotic complications, such as deep vein thrombosis and cerebral infarction. More recently much milder forms of the disease have become apparent, presenting with vascular disease at times of stress to the metabolic pathway involved, which is folate and pyridoxine dependent, for example, during pregnancy (Newman and Mitchell 1984).

The heterozygous state among people under 50 years old is associated with a 10-fold increased risk of cerebral infarction (Beors *et al.* 1985), and if this finding can be replicated among a more typical group of patients, may be a very important risk factor as the heterozygous state is very common, affecting about 1 in 70 of the population. Moreover, a high proportion of people with the homozygous state respond to treatment with pyridoxine, but whether the apparent increased risk in heterozygotes can be treated in the same way is not known.

Variation in time

Stroke mortality rates have shown a consistent decline in several countries (Anon. 1983). In the United States, the rate of decline has been about 0.5 per cent per year from 1900 to 1920, 1 per cent per year from 1920 to 1950, about 1.5 per cent per year from 1950 to 1970, and about 4–5 per cent per year from 1974 onwards (Ostfeld 1980; Whisnant 1984). Data from England and Wales also show a similar decline from 1964, affecting all age groups. These changes are unlikely to have been caused by changes in diagnostic fashion (e.g. a tendency to diagnose myocardial infarction rather than stroke), although attempts to distinguish between time trends in cerebral haemorrhage and infarction (Acheson and Sanderson

1978) are beset with problems of diagnostic accuracy and fashion, and are not reliable.

It is possible that improved survival after a stroke has led to a decline in mortality rates, and evidence from hospital series suggests that case fatality has dropped by about 30 per cent from 1955 to 1971(Haberman *et al.* 1978). However, case fatality might have fallen because of a trend of less severe stroke patients being admitted to hospital. The experience of a whole population has been examined and reduced case fatality confirmed over time (Garraway *et al.* 1983*a*). However, long-term survival for seven years after a stroke has increased much more (by 82 per cent) than one-month survival (by 11 per cent) from 1945–49 to 1970–74. This very modest improvement in early case fatality makes it much more likely that declining incidence rather than reduced case fatality is the explanation for reduced mortality rates, as early deaths greatly outweigh later deaths.

The first reports of a decline in the incidence of stroke were from Rochester, USA, where using the same diagnostic criteria from 1945–1971, a fall of almost 2 per cent per year was found (Garraway *et al.* 1979). Similar falls in incidence have been reported from Japan (Tanaka *et al.* 1981; Ueda *et al.* 1981), and from Finland (Tuomilehto *et al.* 1986). In Sweden, although mortality has fallen, it has been claimed that no parallel decline in incidence has occurred (Alfredsson *et al.* 1986). This discrepancy is probably because only patients admitted to hospital were considered when measuring incidence and the time span was from 1974 to 1981. The study did find that cerebral haemorrhage incidence had declined by almost 2 per cent and 6 per cent per year for men and women respectively. It is quite possible that increased reporting of symptoms of stroke and increased use of neuro-radiology led to higher ascertainment of cases, and thus an increased overall incidence over this relatively short time period. However, increased use of CT scanning might be expected to lead to more diagnoses of cerebral haemorrhage, rather than the fall observed.

Recent incidence trends in Rochester, USA have also shown an increase (Broderick *et al.* 1989). In 1980–84 the incidence of stroke was 17 per cent higher than in 1975–79. This has happened despite better and more vigorous treatment for high blood pressure. The most obvious explanation is that increased investigation of patients, and particularly elderly people, has led to detection of milder cases.

Formerly, such cases might have remained undiagnosed. This is supported by the fall in case fatality for stroke which has dropped from 33 per cent in 1945–49 to only 17 per cent in 1980–84.

Why should incidence of stroke decline?

Four main reasons can be put forward: treatment of high blood pressure; reduced exposure to risk factors associated with high blood pressure; reduced exposure to other risk factors for stroke; and the competing risk of ischaemic heart disease.

Treatment. Treatment of high blood pressure is an extremely implausible explanation for a trend that began in 1900 before any effective anti-hypertensive therapy was available. Treatment has been put forward as the major explanation and the earlier trends have been discounted because incidence data was not available to 'confirm the mortality trend' (Whisnant 1984). Widespread use of acceptable and effective drugs did not begin until the 1960s (Ostfeld 1980; Acheson and Williams 1980; Haberman *et al.* 1978), and while treatment may be a good explanation for the greater rate of decline observed in the 1970s (Tuomilehto *et al.* 1985; Nicholls and Johansen 1983) it would be necessary to make assumptions about the effectiveness of anti-hypertensive treatment that are unlikely. Bonita and Beaglehole (1986) showed that if all hypertensives were treated, and treatment was as effective as in the major published trials, only 10 per cent of the observed reduction in deaths among people aged between 30 and 69 could be explained by treatment. Moreover, older people have experienced just as great a reduction in stroke risk, yet anti-hypertensive treatment was probably much less often given to the aged.

Changes in risk factors associated with high blood pressure. Reduced salt intake over the last century has been put forward as an explanation for a reduced prevalence of high blood pressure, and hence a lower risk of stroke (Joosens *et al.* 1979; Walker 1977; Simpson 1979; Cummins 1983). This presupposes that salt is linked with blood pressure, but evidence from the Intersalt Project was equivocal (Intersalt Cooperative Research Group 1988). Variation in blood pressure between participating centres was not linked with urinary sodium excretion, although there was a weak link between salt excretion and blood pressure within centres. However, it is still possible that a time trend of declining blood pressure might be explained by lowered salt intake. To do this it is necessary to postulate that intakes early this century were extremely high and that a threshold effect on blood pressure operates. Present salt intakes are now below this threshold and consequently no relationship is found now between salt and blood pressure.

The shape of the blood pressure curve in populations may have shifted downwards during this century. Svanborg (1988), in a series of cohort studies, has shown that the mean systolic pressure of people born in 1901/2 at age 70 was 168 mm Hg, whereas people born 10 years later had mean pressures of 162 mm Hg at age 70. A small shift to the left of the population distribution of blood pressure may have a disproportionately great effect on the incidence of stroke (Rose 1981), and is discussed further in this chapter (Attributable risk, p. 24).

Exposure to other risk factors. Major changes in cigarette consumption, physical activity, and diet occurred in the 1970s, which may be much more important determinants of the recent reduction in risk of stroke than treatment of high blood pressure. Among North Americans who adopted a 'healthy life style' earlier than the British, ischaemic heart disease risk started to fall sooner than in Britain. It is possible that the shared risk factors between stroke and ischaemic heart disease operate with a different latency; reductions in shared risk factors may have a more immediate effect on stroke than myocardial infarction.

The association between atmospheric pollution and stroke mortality time trends (Knox 1981) may be an important determinant as it would explain variations in stroke risk in the north and south of Britain, and also social class gradients of risk.

Competing risk of ischaemic heart disease. It has been suggested that stroke-prone individuals have been dying from ischaemic heart disease, and therefore are not surviving to an age when they would have a stroke (Haberman *et al.* 1982). However, stroke mortality rates have fallen more amongst people aged 45–64 years for whom it is more difficult to postulate such an effect on survival.

Variation in place

Studies of geographical variation in stroke incidence have been reviewed (Malmgren *et al.* 1987) and major deficiencies in study design highlighted:

(1) changing criteria for diagnosis;

(2) poor ascertainment of cases;

(3) defining the population at risk;

(4) inadequate size of study;

(5) study of only a few months rather than complete years;

(6) non-standard presentation of rates by age group and sex.

Because of these study defects and other differences between studies it is impossible to decide whether stroke is more or less common in different parts of the world, or whether incidence is truly declining. This is overstating the case and evidence from the WHO multicentre study (Aho *et al.* 1980) and from a carefully conducted incidence study in Japan (Tanaka *et al.* 1981) support the notion that the risk of stroke is higher in Japan than in the United States or United Kingdom. Studies of migrants also support the idea that different populations differ in their risk of stroke (Bonita *et al.* 1984; Kagan *et al.* 1979).

The use of information about variation in place is that it may give clues to aetiology, but interpretation of differences between countries is as difficult as the interpretation of time trends, and is a weak method of testing aetiological hypotheses because so many factors differ between countries. It is, however, a useful method of trying to detect differences in stroke risk due to potential risk factors that are so ubiquitous in a single population (e.g. air pollution, salt intake) that contrasting groups for comparison cannot be found. It is thought likely that most of the variation between countries is a reflection of differences in blood pressure, lipids, and glucose tolerance (Christie 1981), to which could be added many of the factors known to be important from studies of risk factors within populations. Unless other plausible risk factors can be identified it is difficult to support a view that further international comparative studies should be mounted in the hope that 'something might turn up'.

Variation within populations

Major risk factors for stroke

Many factors appear to influence the chance of having a stroke: male sex; increased age; high blood pressure; smoking; body build; alcohol; ischaemic heart disease and atrial fibrillation; previous transient ischaemic attacks; diabetes; lower social class; raised lipids; polycythaemia; physical inactivity; various medication (anti-hypertensives, oestrogens); diet; place of residence; climate; and air quality (Kannel and Wolf 1983). The magnitude of some of these associations is shown in Table 1.3.

Early studies appeared to have underestimated the effects of smoking on risk of stroke (Dawber 1980). Subsequent re-analysis of the Framingham data has found a two-fold increased risk associated with smoking, with a dose response relationship, after allowing for other major risk factors (Wolf *et al.* 1988). The role of alcohol has also only recently been recognized despite its known relationship with blood pressure (Klatsky *et al.* 1977; Saunders 1987). The risks of acute intoxication appear to have a direct effect on risk of stroke, but long term intake may also have an effect independent of blood pressure (Gill *et al.* 1986).

Oral contraceptive use is strongly associated with risk of cerebral thrombosis, but not with haemorrhage. Early studies linking oral contraceptive use with sub-arachnoid haemorrhage were probably due to a link between oral contraceptives and raised blood pressure. The very high risks of myocardial infarction among older contraceptive users who also smoke do not seem to apply to stroke (Sartwell and Stolley 1982).

Most studies have only considered the risk factors for all types of stroke combined, or for clinically classified thrombotic stroke. In general case control studies tend to comprise patients with cerebral thrombosis or embolism because of survival bias (those with cerebral haemorrhage are more likely to die), and because in most countries cerebral thrombosis is more common than cerebral haemorrhage, relative risk estimates are weighted towards describing the risk factors of thrombotic events. A Japanese study examining risk factors for cerebral haemorrhage (defined clinically and with blood stained CSF on lumbar puncture) found that raised blood pressure, high alcohol intake and high cholesterol level were all strong risk factors (Tanaka *et al.* 1982).

Table 1.3 Risk factors for stroke

Risk factor	*Relative risk*	*Source*
Age (55–64 vs. 75 +)	5	Oxfordshire Community Stroke Project (1983)
Blood pressure (160/95 + vs. <120/80)	7	Dawber (1980)
Smoking (current status)	4;* 3; 2	Salonen *et al.* (1982); Bonita (1986); Wolf *et al.* (1988)
Body build (3 kg/m² increase; obesity)	1; 1.8	MRC (1988); Herman *et al.* (1983)
Ischaemic heart disease	2.9; 3	Herman *et al.* (1982*b*); Kannel *et al.* (1983)
Heart failure	5	Kannel *et al.* (1983)
Atrial fibrillation	3.5; 5.6; 6.9	Herman *et al.* (1982*b*); Wolf *et al.* (1978); Flegel *et al.* (1987)
Past TIA	5.2	Herman *et al.* (1982*b*)
Diabetes mellitus	2.2	Herman *et al.* (1982*b*); Kannel *et al.* (1983)
Social class (I vs. V)	1.6	Acheson and Sanderson (1978)
Blood triglycerides (6.5 mmol/l +)	2.4*	Salonen *et al.* (1982)
Raised haematocrit		Kannel *et al.* (1972); Tohgi *et al.* (1978)
Physical activity (little vs. light/heavy	2.5	Herman *et al.* (1982*b*)
Oral contraceptives (ever used)	9	Sartwell and Stolley (1982)
Postmenopausal oestrogens	0.53	Paganini-Hill *et al.* (1988)
Alcohol (acute intoxication)	5*	Syrjanen *et al.* (1988); Gill *et al.* (1986); Hillbohm and Kaste (1983)

* Men only.

Other risk factors

Diet. This may have a causative role in stroke. An association has been found between a high dietary intake of potassium (derived from 24-hour dietary recall reports) and subsequent deaths from stroke in a longitudinal study of people aged 50 to 79 and followed for 12 years (Khaw and Barrett-Connor 1987). In this study, a 10 mmol daily increase in dietary potassium was associated with a 40 per cent reduction in risk of stroke death. This association was substantiated when adjustment was made for hypertension (in itself associated with a low potassium intake), age, sex, obesity, smoking, and blood glucose. A weaker, although still statistically significant relationship with morbidity was found, and the authors commented that the association may reflect an effect of potassium on stroke survival rather than on incidence.

These observations link with data on stroke mortality and consumption of vitamin C-containing foods which are also potassium-rich (Acheson and Williams 1983). A correlation exists between regional stroke mortality rates in England and Scotland and regional consumption of vitamin C-containing green vegetables and fruit obtained from National Food Survey data. There are plausible pathogenetic mechanisms (capillary fragility, reduced platelet adhesiveness) that might explain an effect on haemorrhagic stroke, and the effect of potassium on hypertension might explain a lowered thrombotic tendency. The correlations observed were high but as the authors acknowledged, this sort of information is a weak method of detecting and testing causal relationships.

Ecological fallacy. The association may well be an example of an ecological fallacy. Whenever a disease varies in time or between places it is obvious to look for factors that also vary between times or places. Such factors may have nothing to do with the risk of disease and to assume that they do is to make a false presumption—an ecological fallacy. In this case, the difference in stroke mortality follows a north-south pattern, with the highest rates in the north. Unfortunately, many other factors also follow this same north-south distribution, and to find an association between one such factor (consumption of fresh green vegetables and fruit) and stroke does not imply causation. Similar correlations might be found between low stroke mortality and a high rate of car ownership, or some other indicator of socio-economic advantage. It is necessary to confirm the relationship at the level of individuals as well as populations before the association can be suspected of being causal.

Our own attempts to test this hypothesis using a case control method, and measuring vitamin C levels by dietary recall and white cell vitamin C assay did not show an association between vitamin C and risk of stroke (Barer *et al.* 1989). In part this may have been because of difficulty in measuring usual vitamin C levels and intake after a stroke has occurred. Khaw's observations (Khaw and Barrett-Connor 1987) using a longitudinal design are a much more powerful method of testing the hypothesis. The next step would be to set up a population experiment in which subjects were supplemented with either potassium and/or vitamin C which would provide the best evidence to confirm or refute a causal link.

Febrile illness. This condition (respiratory infection in 80 per cent of cases) in the month prior to onset was associated with a nine-fold increased risk of ischaemic stroke among patients under the age of 50 in a case control study (Syrjanen *et al.* 1988). The mechanism for this association is not clear, and was not due to bacterial endocarditis and septic emboli. The authors commented on the possibility of upper respiratory tract infections causing 'local inflammatory arteritis of the carotid' and of possible immune complex mediated vasculitis and platelet aggregation. Another possibility that was not considered is that these young patients were predisposed to thrombosis through being heterozygous for homocystinuria, and the infection was sufficient stimulus for a thrombosis to occur. The strength of this association is very high and consequently merits further study.

Cold stress. Seasonal variation in risk of dying from stroke has been reported (Haberman *et al.* 1981) which may be due to an effect on survival after suffering a stroke or a direct effect on incidence. However, in Australia, stroke incidence has been shown to closely parallel ambient temperature (Christie 1981), and in Nottingham a significant negative correlation between air temperature and numbers of patients admitted to hospital with an acute stroke two days later was found (Barer *et al.* 1984). Paradoxically admissions to hospital in Carlisle, England, peaked in the summer months (Chin *et al.* 1980), although the differences reported could be explained by chance variation, or differences in the age structure of the population at risk during the summer, or a tendency for older people having strokes to be admitted to hospital because relatives are away on holiday during the summer.

Cold causes both a rise in blood pressure (Brennan *et al.* 1982), and an increase in blood viscosity (Keatinge *et al.* 1984) which together might explain the increased risk of stroke associated with cold weather. Unfortunately, the simple measure of central heating for old people at greatest risk does not produce any change in their seasonal mortality pattern (Keatinge 1986), although specific effects on stroke incidence have not been measured.

Risk factors among older people

Much of the research quoted did not study the people most at risk of stroke—those aged over 75. The importance of some risk factors seems to decline with age, in particular hypertension (Mattila *et al.* 1988; Evans *et al.* 1980; Evans 1979; Evans 1987). Evans' study of the population of Newcastle is surprising because although only 16 per cent were over 80 years no relationship between blood pressure and risk of stroke was found. Evans' study however confirmed that a history of previous high blood pressure, intermittent claudication, use of drugs to treat heart failure and symptoms of vascular disease, ECG abnormalities, and above average estimated weight for height at age 25 were associated with similar levels of increased risk as among younger populations.

A study of stroke patients aged from 65 to 75 demonstrated that hypertension, diabetes mellitus, and a past history of myocardial infarction were as strongly associated with stroke in this age band as at younger ages (Himmelman *et al.* 1988). Large prospective studies examining the effects of risk factors among older people have not been done. Despite the weakening of the association between hypertension and stroke among elderly people, the two trials of anti-hypertensives in older people both showed a positive benefit of treating old people (Amery *et al.* 1985; Coope and Warrender 1986). The benefits (if any) of treatment in very old age (over 80 years) remain unclear. The relationships between other risk factors and stroke in the high seventies and eighties also remain unanswered.

Which risk factors are most important?

This question can be examined in three ways:

(1) which risk factors are most strongly associated with risk of stroke;

(2) which risk factors are treatable;

(3) which risk factors are 'responsible for' (or explain) the largest numbers of strokes?

Strength of association

Table 1.3 shows the strength of association in terms of relative risk of stroke, given the presence of each risk factor. Age, heart failure, atrial fibrillation, past TIA, and acute alcohol intoxication all look very important with relative risks of five-fold or more. Relative risk has the disadvantage that the baseline risk for comparison has a major effect on the magnitude of the relative risk. For example, blood pressure could be made to look more important by altering the criterion used from 160/95 + to a systolic pressure of 180 + mmHg, which has a relative risk of eight-fold when compared with people whose systolic pressures are below 120 mmHg.

Treatability

Blood pressure, smoking, obesity, diabetes, inactivity, heart disease, atrial fibrillation, transient ischaemic attacks, polycythaemia, alcohol abuse, and raised blood lipids might be considered treatable. The benefits of treating blood pressure even at mildly raised levels have been demonstrated (MRC 1985). The use of aspirin after TIA and mild stroke is probably of benefit in preventing further TIAs and strokes (see Chapter 8) (Antiplatelet Trialists' Collaboration 1988). Treatment with beta-blockade after myocardial infarction is associated with improved survival (Mitchell 1982) and vasodilators improve the prognosis for survival in patients with heart failure (Cohn *et al.* 1986). It is possible that such treatments will reduce the risk of subsequent stroke, although this has not been conclusively documented. Treatment of diabetes, polycythaemia, and atrial fibrillation are not of proven benefit in reducing the risk of stroke. Smoking, obesity, alcohol abuse, and inactivity are all behaviours that should be modified for many reasons, but on present evidence perhaps only smoking can be singled out as being justified on the basis of reducing the risk of stroke (MRC 1988; Bonita *et al.* 1986).

Attributable risk

This is an important concept because it allows for both the strength with which a risk factor is associated with a disease, and the commonness of the risk factor. A strong risk factor (e.g. acute alcohol intoxication) may only affect a small proportion of the population and therefore be 'responsible for' only a very small number of strokes. The stronger the risk factor and the more common, the larger is its attributable risk. It is always important to remember that association does not mean causation, and when thinking about attributable risk it is easy to fall into the trap of assuming that because a high proportion of a disease may be attributed to a particular risk factor, that removing that risk factor would lead to a commensurate fall in the occurrence of the disease.

Blood pressure provides a good example of the relationship between high relative risk but low attributable risk. Table 1.4 shows how dramatically the incidence of stroke rises with blood pressure. However the proportion of people with blood pressures over 180 mmHg is small, although their relative risk of having a stroke is 31.8/1.7 = 18.7 times higher than people with pressures below 120 mmHg. The expected number of cases of stroke associated with each blood pressure stratum obviously depends on the

Table 1.4 The relationship between risk of stroke among men aged 40–49 and the expected number of cases arising in each blood pressure stratum over 24 years, using data from the Framingham study (Dawber 1980)

Systolic BP	*Prevalence* (%)	Incidence rate/100/24 yrs	Expected no. of cases (%)	
<120	16	1.7	27	(4.7)
120–	43	3.6	155	(27.0)
140–	29	5.6	162	(28.3)
160–	8	12.8	102	(17.8)
180+	4	31.8	127	(22.2)
	100		573	(100.0)

numbers at risk. The expected numbers of strokes occurring at each level is calculated by multiplying the percentage prevalence of people in a particular blood pressure level by the incidence rate for that level. People with pressures over 180 mmHg constitute only 22.2 per cent of all the cases that might be expected to occur, and even those who might be considered hypertensive (+160 mmHg) only comprise about 40 per cent of the total cases in this population of men aged 40–49. Thus, although blood pressure is important in terms of its relative risk, its attributable risk is not so pronounced.

The implication is that treatment which aims to lower high blood pressure can have only a limited effect in reducing the number of cases of stroke in a whole community. If, for example, treatment of people with systolic blood pressures over 160 mmHg produced a 25 per cent reduction in strokes, or even a 50 per cent reduction, the overall benefits would be quite modest in terms of the reduction in the numbers of strokes. This is shown in Table 1.5. Even on the assumption of a 50 per cent reduction in incidence rates, treatment produces only a 20 per cent reduction in the total numbers of strokes that might be expected. Bonita and Beaglehole (1986), when estimating whether treatment of high blood pressure might have contributed to the reduction in stroke mortality, estimated that only a 10 per cent reduction could be attributed to treatment.

Table 1.5 The effects of treatment assuming a reduction in incidence of 25% and 50% for people with blood pressures over 160 mmHg, using data from Table 1.4

Systolic BP	*Prevalence (%)*	*25% reduction*		*50% reduction*	
		Incidence rate	*Expected cases*	*Incidence rate*	*Expected cases*
<120	16	1.7	27	1.7	27
120–	43	3.6	155	3.6	155
140–	29	5.6	162	5.6	162
160–	8	9.6	77	6.4	51
180+	4	23.9	96	15.9	64
			517		459

i.e. $(573-517)/573\times 100=10\%$. $(573-459)/573\times 100=20\%$.

Rose (1981) has drawn attention to this apparent paradox that high risk approaches to disease control, that is searching for those with the highest levels of risk factors and treating them as actively as possible, can only contribute a small amount to population control of disease. Rose estimated that a small downward shift in the population distribution of blood pressure of as little as 2–3 mmHg might be associated with as much reduction in mortality as drug treatment for those at high risk. This effect of shifting the blood pressure distribution downward is shown in Table 1.6. The total number of cases expected is 90 per cent of the total expected with the original blood pressure distribution, an effect of the same size as achieved by a treatment that reduces the risk of stroke by 25 per cent, demonstrated in Table 1.5.

Svanborg's observations (1988) that systolic blood pressures have fallen among successive birth cohorts since the beginning of this century suggest that this downward shift phenomenon is actually happening. Quite why this has happened and whether further cohorts will be affected remains to be seen.

The attributable risk describes the proportion of disease that is associated with exposure to that particular risk factor. It can be calculated from either rate ratio or odds ratio estimates of the relative risk, and the proportion of the population exposed to the risk factor. This latter measure can be taken directly from population-based cohort studies where the proportion exposed is known. In case control studies, the proportion exposed in the control group

Table 1.6 The effect of a small downward shift in the distribution of systolic blood pressure (per cent prevalence) on the expected number of strokes, using data from Table 1.4

Systolic BP	*Prevalence* (%)	Incidence rate/100/24 yrs	Expected no. of cases
<120	17	1.7	29
120–	44	3.6	158
140–	26	5.6	146
160–	7	12.8	90
180+	3	31.8	95
	100		518 (90%)

may not be a good estimate of the true level of exposure in the population, particularly if the controls were selected from hospital admissions (where cigarette smokers will be over-represented for example) or if matching between cases and controls was used in the study design. It may be necessary to make estimates of the proportion of the population exposed from other studies, or routine surveys. The mathematical relationship between attributable risk and relative risk is:

$$\text{Attributable risk} = \frac{P \times (RR - 1)}{P \times (RR - 1) + 1}$$

where P is the proportion of the population exposed and RR is the relative risk estimate. Figure 1.1 shows the relationship for a series of different relative risks and proportions of the population exposed to the risk factor.

Applying this relationship to some of the risk factors for stroke suggests that some factors such as physical inactivity, despite relatively low relative risks, affect so many people that their contribution to the population burden of disease may be substantial. For

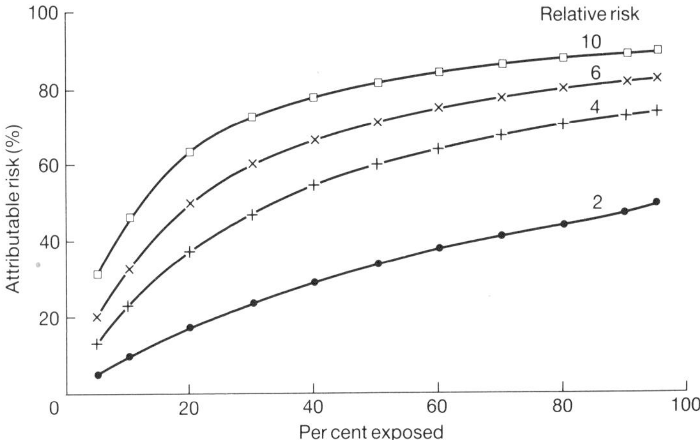

Fig. 1.1 Attributable risk, relative risk, and the proportion of the population exposed to a risk factor. For example, if a risk factor (such as lack of exercise) has a relative risk of 2, and 80% of the population have this risk factor, then 45% of strokes can be attributed to this risk factor. Note that attributing strokes to a risk factor does not mean that removing the risk factor would result in a commensurate reduction in strokes.

example, if 60 per cent of the population are inactive, and the relative risk of stroke amongst such people is 2.5-fold, applying the formula:

$$\text{Attributable risk} = \frac{0.6 \times (2.5 - 1)}{0.6 \times (2.5 - 1) + 1} = 47.4\%$$

This implies that almost half of all strokes may be attributed to inactivity. The attributable risks of smoking and high blood pressure were found to be of comparable size (about a third of strokes associated with each) in a New Zealand study (Bonita *et al.* 1986).

By contrast, a past history of transient ischaemic attack affects less than 1 per cent of the population (Sandercock and Warlow 1985), so despite its high relative risk of 5, less than 2 per cent of the stroke burden can be attributed to this cause. Looking for effective treatments for TIAs should therefore be put into some perspective by this information. Even if a remarkable treatment was discovered that prevented every single case of stroke following TIA, it would only lead to a reduction in the overall numbers of strokes of less than 2 per cent. Similar comments apply to the presence of heart failure, diabetes mellitus, and atrial fibrillation, which only affect relatively small proportions of younger people. Among older people, however, the prevalence of heart disease is much higher, with up to 15 per cent with some sort of 'heart trouble' (Evans *et al.* 1980). The attributable risks of some risk factors may become more important in terms of their contribution to the overall burden of disease despite becoming weaker in terms of their relative risk.

The importance of this approach is that it gives an idea of where effort might usefully be made to prevent disease or look for new treatments. Thus, although around half of all strokes may be associated with physical inactivity, it is not known whether increased activity will lead to a reduction in risk of strokes. Attributable risk estimates are not a substitute for trials to estimate the true effects of interventions.

Summary

1. Estimates of the risk of having a stroke can be obtained from both case control and longitudinal studies. In the former case, the odds ratio is a reasonable approximation of the ratio of incidence

rates in exposed and non-exposed groups, provided the incidence rates are low.

2. Family and twin studies suggest that early influences in life (intra-uterine or within-family environment) may have an impact on subsequent risk of stroke. Such influences may be mediated through blood pressure, although an independent family effect is probable.

3. The decline in stroke mortality is due to a decline in incidence, and the factors responsible may include a downward shift in the population distribution of blood pressure, and changes in other factors that may influence the frequency of stroke, such as atmospheric pollution and diet. Treatment of high blood pressure can explain only about 10% of the decline.

4. Blood pressure, age, smoking, heart failure, transient ischaemic attack, acute alcohol intoxication, and atrial fibrillation all increase the relative risk of stroke by several-fold.

5. The importance of risk factors is best assessed by considering not only the size of the relative risk, but also the proportion of the population exposed to the risk factor, using the attributable risk. Risk factors with high attributable risks are primary targets for trials of prevention and treatment.

6. About a third of all strokes may be attributed to raised blood pressure and a third to smoking. Physical inactivity may be associated with a high attributable risk because of its commonness. Attributing a proportion of stroke occurrence to a particular factor does not mean that removing that factor would lead to a reduction in the numbers of strokes by the same proportion. Clinical trials remain the best method of determining whether changing a risk factor reduces the occurrence of disease.

2 Diagnosis

Strokes are caused by arteriovascular events: thrombosis; haemorrhage; and emboli. However, not all patients who present with signs and symptoms of hemiplegia have had a stroke. The nomenclature used to describe patients can lead to problems, in particular calling all patients with signs suggestive of a stroke a 'CVA' or cerebrovascular accident. By using CVA the implication is that a stroke has occurred and no further pathological processes need to be ruled out. The term CVA can also cause confusion because it may refer to the side of the lesion or the side of the signs.

Strokes must be separated from other diseases that mimic stroke because the treatment and prognosis are often different. Within the category of stroke, it is now increasingly important to distinguish haemorrhage from thrombosis and emboli because anti-platelet agents are increasingly used for the latter, but may be hazardous for the former group. For research purposes (e.g. describing natural history, evaluating treatments) it is desirable to deal with homogeneous pathological entities so that potentially useful information about haemorrhage or lacunae is not lost in the majority of thromboses.

Diagnosis of stroke

A stroke is a focal or global neurological impairment of sudden onset, lasting more than 24 hours (or leading to death), and of presumed vascular aetiology (WHO 1978). The commonness of stroke may encourage diagnostic laziness but it is important to remember that the hemiplegic syndrome may have many causes. Some of these causes may lead to an increased tendency to thrombosis, embolism, or haemorrhage; others may produce a hemiplegic stroke syndrome but not through a vascular pathogenetic mechanism. The doctor's first task when seeing a patient with a focal or global neurological impairment is to decide whether the symptoms and signs are caused by a vascular lesion or not. It is tempting to assume that if a patient has a typical history and signs of hemiplegia then the probability of the diagnosis being vascular stroke is certain.

To measure the accuracy of clinical diagnosis comparison with some 'gold standard' is necessary. Autopsy evidence is often taken to be the best indicator of the presence or absence of a pathological lesion, and comparisons with clinical diagnosis have been made by Heasman and Lipworth (1966). These authors attempted to examine the accuracy of diagnosis in as unselected a series of cases as possible, and the autopsy rates were substantially higher than usual during the period of their study. A total of 9501 autopsy diagnoses were compared with the final clinical diagnoses from which it is possible to calculate the sensitivity and specificity (that is the accuracy) of clinical diagnosis of stroke, which is shown in Table 2.1.

These estimates of accuracy may be inflated because they are only relevant to those patients who died and therefore had severe and probably more obvious symptoms and signs. It is possible that clinical diagnosis is less accurate when the symptoms and signs are less severe. However, it is likely that clinical diagnosis is more accurate now than in the 1950s because of increased use of neuroradiology for patients with atypical presentations.

Sensitivity and specificity are not indicators of accuracy of diagnosis that appeal to clinicians' intuition. Clinicians do not know what the autopsy result is or will be, but only their own

Table 2.1 The accuracy of final clinical diagnosis of stroke from 'not stroke' using autopsy findings as the diagnostic standard (from Heasman and Lipworth 1966)

Final clinical diagnosis	*Autopsy diagnosis*		
	Stroke	*Not stroke*	
Stroke	820	276	1096
Not stroke	92	8313	8405
Total	912	8589	9501

Sensitivity of clinical diagnosis 820/912: 90%.
Specificity of clinical diagnosis 8313/8589: 97%.

diagnosis. In other words, their experience of accuracy is derived from the rows of tables such as Table 2.1 and not from the columns (i.e. sensitivity and specificity). Clinicians are rightly interested in the extent to which they will be correct if they say the patient has a stroke (i.e. positive predictive value), and the opposite of this, how often they will be wrong when they think a patient does not have a stroke (i.e. negative predictive value). Using Heasman and Lipworth's data, the clinician will be correct in the diagnosis of stroke 75 per cent of the time (i.e. 820/1096) and correct in not diagnosing a stroke 99 per cent of the time (i.e. 8313/8405). This fits in with intuition; doctors do not often miss a stroke because the signs are so obvious, but there are other causes of these signs which may lead to a false-positive diagnosis of a cerebrovascular accident.

Elderly people are most likely to suffer from misdiagnosis of stroke. This may be because of their relatively non-specific presentation (i.e. confusion, incontinence, immobility) when acutely ill, and multiple pathology. These factors make it harder to distinguish, for example, whether an exacerbation of bronchitis has led to increased weakness from an old stroke, or whether a new stroke has occurred. The accuracy of clinical diagnosis might be improved by training, relating the clinical signs detected with neuro-radiological and autopsy examinations, by increased monitoring of progress of patients, and by better knowledge of the natural history of stroke.

Differentiating stroke from other diseases

More typically the problem for doctors is to distinguish non-vascular from vascular (i.e. thrombosis, haemorrhage, or embolism) causes of neurological impairment. Several studies have examined this question and are summarized in Table 2.2.

The variability of these estimates of diagnostic accuracy are surprising at first sight. Part of the explanation may be the type of patients studied. Older patients may have a higher risk of non-vascular pathology (e.g. subdural haematoma, cerebral abscess, cerebral metastases, iatrogenic hypoglycaemia, etc.), which will lead to more false-positive diagnoses of stroke and thus a lower specificity of clinical diagnosis. Allen (1983) excluded any patient over 75 years which may explain why the specificity found was so high.

Another explanation is the skill of the clinician. Norris and

Table 2.2 Accuracy of diagnosis of stroke from other causes of neurological impairment

Source	*'Gold standard'*	*Sensitivity (%)*	*Specificity (%)*
Allen (1983)	CT scan + autopsy	67	91
Heasman and Lipworth (1966)	Autopsy	80	-
Norris and Hachinski (1982)	CT scan + autopsy	100	22–76
Weisberg and Nice (1977)	CT scan	72	76
Hatano (1976)	Autopsy	99	69

Hachinski (1982) examined the effect of the doctor's experience in some detail. They asked junior emergency room doctors, neurology residents, and neurology consultants to assess 93 autopsy-proven stroke patients for four items of information: stroke present or not; ischaemic or haemorrhagic pathogenesis; right- or left-sided lesion; and hemisphere or brainstem lesion. From these they derived an 'accuracy' score by adding up correct answers so that the maximum score a doctor could get was 372 (i.e. 93 × 4). They demonstrated that consultants were the most accurate (89 per cent), neurology residents did not do badly (77 per cent), and that junior emergency room doctors had a lot to learn (38 per cent).

Norris and Hachinski (1982) also looked at the question of the specificity of clinical diagnosis, that is how often doctors were correct when they *ruled out* a diagnosis of a stroke clinically. They examined the diagnoses of the same groups of doctors among a consecutive series of 50 patients admitted to their unit as stroke patients but who subsequently turned out not to have had a stroke. The junior emergency room doctors gave a correct diagnosis of 'not stroke' in 22 per cent, neurology residents in 32 per cent, and consultants in 76 per cent of cases.

The frequency of misdiagnosis, or the predictive value of a positive diagnosis (i.e. 1 – misdiagnosis rate) of stroke is often reported (Heasman and Lipworth 1966; Norris and Hachinski, 1982; Allen 1983; Sandercock *et al.* 1985*a*) but is not a very useful figure because it depends on the frequency of other non-stroke diagnoses among the patients studied. Reference to Table 2.3 may help to explain this. Although accuracy of diagnosis remains the same, altering the proportion of strokes to non-strokes will have a major effect on the positive and negative predictive values. For example, Norris and Hachinski (1982) found that 108 (13 per cent) out of 821 consecutive patients initially thought to have a stroke turned out to have some other pathology. Whereas, the Oxford Community Stroke Study (Sandercock *et al.* 1985*a*) only found five (1.5 per cent) out of 325 first strokes with unsuspected nonvascular pathology. As the commonest reason for misdiagnosis in Norris and Hachinski's study was *grand mal* fits occurring in patients who had had a previous stroke it is not surprising that their estimate of misdiagnosis was so much higher than the Oxford group who only considered first events, excluding those with previous strokes.

The mode of onset of a stroke is thought to be an indicator of nonvascular pathology and Allen (1983) demonstrated that a stuttering or progressively evolving onset of the stroke was more often associated with a 'mass' lesion (i.e. tumour or subdural haematoma). The sensitivity and specificity of a stuttering onset for mass lesions were 56 and 80 per cent respectively but was associated with only a 14 per cent predictive value; i.e. for every 100 patients suspected of having a mass lesion rather than a stroke because of a stuttering onset, the doctor would be wrong in 86 cases and correct in 14 cases. This level of detection would not please a neuro-radiologist performing CT brain scans for this indication. Weisberg and Nice (1977) found very similar results in a comparison of patients suffering a sudden onset with those whose onset was not sudden. Allen (1983) drew attention to the sensitivity of a poor history as an indicator of a mass lesion, but in this case too, its predictive value was low—13 per cent.

It is quite possible that two doctors can be equally accurate (i.e. same sensitivity and specificity) in their clinical diagnosis of stroke but have very different 'misdiagnosis' (or predictive value) rates. Table 2.3 shows how this can happen. The low frequency of vascular pathology might represent the practice of a primary health care or emergency room doctor. The high frequency of vascular pathology might be what is seen by a neurologist in a tertiary referral hospital specializing in difficult cases. In both high and low frequency situations the accuracy of diagnosis is assumed to be the same: sensitivity 90 per cent, specificity 90 per cent.

This relationship between predictive value and frequency of the

Table 2.3 The relationship between frequency of nonvascular pathology causing neurological impairment and predictive value of clinical diagnosis

1. *A low frequency of vascular pathology: 1%.*
   Sensitivity 90%; Specificity 90%.

Clinical diagnosis	*True diagnosis*		
	Stroke	*Not stroke*	
Stroke	9	99	108
Not stroke	1	891	892
	10	990	1000

Predictive value of a clinical diagnosis of stroke: 9/108, i.e. 8%.

2. *A high frequency of vascular pathology: 10%.*
   Sensitivity 90%; Specificity 90%.

Clinical diagnosis	*True diagnosis*		
	Stroke	*Not stroke*	
Stroke	90	90	180
Not stroke	10	810	820
	100	900	1000

Predictive value of a clinical diagnosis of stroke: 90/180, i.e. 50%.

disease of interest makes predictive value an unstable, and therefore less useful measure of misdiagnosis or diagnostic accuracy.

Diagnosis of cerebral haemorrhage and infarction

The need to distinguish haemorrhage from thrombo-embolic mechanisms of stroke is gaining much greater importance with increased use of anti-platelet agents (see Chapter 8), and other thrombolytic agents. Within the infarction category, a case has been made for separating lacunar strokes from other types of infarction largely because they form a distinct clinical group which may have a different response to treatment (Bamford and Warlow, 1988).

The predictive value of a clinical diagnosis (i.e. how often a diagnosis is correct) is the most relevant piece of information for assessing the ability to distinguish cerebral haemorrhage from infarction, yet it is affected largely by the frequency of haemorrhage among the patients studied, in the same way that the ability of doctors to pick out nonvascular pathology is more dependent on its frequency than on the clinical accuracy of the doctors (see Table 2.3).

The likelihood ratio

A method of summarizing the accuracy of a diagnosis (or of an investigation or test) is to calculate the likelihood ratio, i.e. the ratio of the proportion of patients who truly have the diagnosis and have a positive clinical diagnosis to the proportion of patients who do *not* really have the diagnosis but have an erroneous positive clinical diagnosis. This is shown in Table 2.4.

The likelihood ratio has some virtues. First it is a single number. More importantly it can be used to calculate easily the predictive value of diagnostic skill (or of an investigation or test) for different frequencies of the disease in the study group. This is because there is a simple relationship between the initial frequency of the disease (before any attempt at diagnosis has been made), the likelihood ratio, and the final probability of the true diagnosis after clinical

Table 2.4 Calculation of the likelihood ratio

Clinical diagnosis	*True diagnosis*	
	Haemorrhage	*Infarction*
Haemorrhage	a	b
Infarction	c	d

Likelihood ratio: Proportion with diagnosis and positive clinical diagnosis (i.e. $a/(a+c)$, i.e. sensitivity) to proportion without diagnosis but with a positive clinical diagnosis (i.e. $b/(b+d)$, i.e. 1 − specificity).
i.e. $[a/(a+c)]/[b/(b+d)]$,
i.e. sensitivity/(1 − specificity).

diagnosis has been made (which is, of course, the predictive value of clinical diagnosis).

For example, if the true frequency of cerebral haemorrhage in a series of stroke patients is 20 per cent (this is often called a 'prior' probability of 0.20), the pre-test odds of haemorrhage are 0.20/(1 – 0.20) which is 0.25. The relationship between probability and odds is:

$$\text{Odds} = \text{Probability}/(1 - \text{Probability}).$$

Multiplying the pre-test odds by the likelihood ratio gives the 'posterior' odds (i.e. in the sense of after attempts at diagnosis) of haemorrhage being truly present. The probability of haemorrhage is then calculated from the relationship:

$$\text{Posterior odds}/(1 + \text{Post-test odds}) = \text{Posterior probability}$$

A full discussion of the calculation of odds, likelihood ratios and probabilities is given by Sackett *et al.* (1985).

An early study (Aring and Merritt 1935) relating autopsy findings with clinical symptoms and signs found that headache at onset, vomiting, neck stiffness, fits, depressed consciousness, high blood pressure at presentation, signs of tentorial herniation, and blood in the CSF were all much more common in patients who had suffered a cerebral haemorrhage than an infarct. There is doubt about the ability of clinicians to diagnose the type of pathology causing a stroke, and Heasman and Lipworth's study (1966) looked at this problem in detail. Their comparison between clinical and autopsy diagnoses is shown in Table 2.5.

They reported their results in terms of predictive values, such as, only 257 (47.7 per cent) out of 539 clinical diagnoses of cerebral haemorrhage were confirmed at autopsy. It is possible to calculate the sensitivity and specificity (and from these, the likelihood ratio) of clinical diagnosis as a means of discriminating between haemorrhage and infarction from their data. The sensitivity is 257/377 (i.e. 68 per cent) and the specificity is 583/865 (i.e. 67 per cent). (The closeness of the two figures is simply a fluke with no significance.)

The likelihood ratio derived from Heasman and Lipworth's data is sensitivity/(1 – specificity) i.e. 0.67/(1 – 0.67) = 2.03. The pre-test probability (or prevalence) of haemorrhage in their series was 377/1242 = 0.30, which is equivalent to pre-test odds of 0.436.

Table 2.5 Comparison between clinical and autopsy diagnoses of type of stroke (from Heasman and Lipworth 1966; table 12, p. 24)

Clinical diagnosis	*Autopsy diagnosis*					
	Haemorrhage	*Thrombosis/ embolism*	*Sub-arachnoid haemorrhage*	*Ill-defined*	*Other causes*	*Total*
Haemorrhage	257 ·	65	40	2	175	539
Thrombosis/ embolism	36	159	3	8	145	351
Sub-arachnoid haemorrhage	34	2	112	–	17	165
Ill-defined	5	8		9	19	41
Other causes	45	76	16	9	–	146
Totals	377	310	171	28	356	1242

Multiplying the pre-test odds by the likelihood ratio gives the post-test odds, which are: $0.436 \times 2.03 = 0.88$.

The post-test odds can then be converted back to a probability (or percentage), which gives $0.88/(1+0.88) = 0.47$ or 47 per cent. In other words, the diagnostic ability of doctors studied in this series was sufficient to increase the probability of a haemorrhage from 30 to 47 per cent. This is the same as the predictive value of a diagnosis of haemorrhage shown in Table 2.3, $257/539 = 47.7$ per cent (the difference is due to rounding errors in the calculations).

All this calculation effort may seem very unnecessary when the predictive value could have been easily calculated in the first place. Likelihood ratios really come into their own when different diagnostic tests are compared, when a series of investigations are used, and strategies for use of invasive or risky investigations have to be planned. The higher the likelihood ratio, the more discriminating is the diagnostic method or test, and hence the more useful. Moreover, the work of converting probabilities to odds can be avoided if a nomogram is used (see Sackett *et al.* 1985).

Likelihood ratios of clinical signs and tests

Other estimates of clinical and test accuracy in diagnosing haemorrhage from infarction have been reported and are summarized in Table 2.6 together with likelihood ratios. In each of these studies the frequency of cerebral haemorrhage varied from half to less than a fifth affected, which would have led to very different estimates of the predictive value of tests or of clinical symptoms and signs. For example, in von Arbin's study, the predictive value of bedside clinical diagnosis was $6/20 = 30$ per cent; whereas Allen (1983) found that his clinical skills in diagnosing haemorrhage gave a predictive value of $14/26 = 54$ per cent, which appears much better. It would be tempting to assume that Allen had superior clinical skills but this would be overlooking the fact that this difference in predictive value is due to the fact that haemorrhage was twice as common in Allen's (18 per cent) as in von Arbin's series of cases (9 per cent), despite both being consecutively selected. The likelihood ratios, however, show that there is little to choose between them.

Another feature of these likelihood ratios for cerebral haemorrhage is that a high value is usually obtained because of a high specificity (i.e. a low false-positive rate). A sign or test that is

Table 2.6 Accuracy of clinical information and tests to diagnose haemorrhage from infarction as the cause of a stroke

Source	*Diagnosis of haemorrhage*		
	Sensitivity (%)	*Specificity (%)*	*Likelihood ratio*
Allen (1983)			
Clinical information	48	91	5.3
Guy's Score method (14+)*	52	98	26.0
Blood stained CSF	50	98	25.0
von Arbin *et al.* (1981)			
Clinical information	33	93	4.7
Impaired consciousness	72	80	3.6
Neck stiffness	28	97	9.3
Britten *et al.* (1983)			
CSF protein > 1G/Litre	89	92	11.1
Xanthochromic CSF	70	95	14.0
Harrison (1980)			
Headache	56	57	1.3
Vomiting	45	93	6.4
Fits at onset	6	91	0.7
Neck stiffness	48	89	4.4
Blood stained CSF	90	100	infinity
Lee *et al.* (1975)			
Bloody/xanthochromic CSF	75	96	18.8

* See Table 2.8.

pathognomonic for a disease must be 100 per cent specific, in other words, it must never occur when the disease is not present. This will give a predictive value of 100 per cent because there are no false-positives, and a likelihood ratio of infinity. So the higher the likelihood ratio the greater the probability the diagnosis (e.g. of cerebral haemorrhage) can be ruled in. A range of likelihood ratios and pre-test probabilities of disease are shown in Fig. 2.1, with the post-test probabilities shown in the body of the figure.

The figure demonstrates how at high pre-test probabilities, even very powerful tests are not able to increase the probability of disease by a great margin. At low disease pre-test probabilities, tests with high likelihood ratios are most useful. However, tests with relatively modest likelihood ratios (in the range 4–10) may be

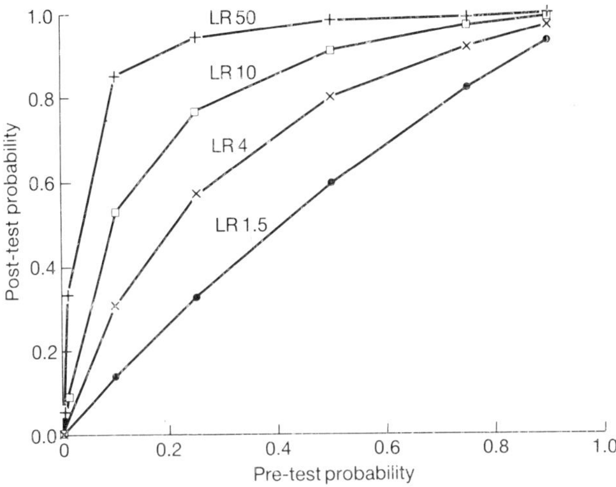

Fig. 2.1 Post-test probabilities of disease following a positive test-result for a range of likelihood ratios and pre-test disease probabilities.

extremely helpful in cases where the pre-test chances of disease being present are around 50 per cent.

Guy's Hospital score

This score (see Table 2.7) depends on obtaining good quality information about the onset of the stroke, the state of the patient at 24 hours and past medical history. For many patients it may be difficult to do this reliably (see Chapter 3 on clinical disagreements). The score is quite simple to use, the presence or absence of symptoms, signs and history are added up (except for diastolic blood pressure—for which the phase and arm taken in were not reported—which is multiplied by a constant and then added to the score). As can be seen, persisting impaired conscious level adds a large component to the score. It would be of value to develop further clinical scoring methods that were less reliant on information that may be difficult to obtain or is often subject to clinical disagreements.

Although Allen (1983) was not very impressed by the extra diagnostic accuracy obtained by use of the scoring method, its

Table 2.7 The Guy's Hospital score for discriminating haemorrhagic from thrombotic stroke (from Allen 1983)

Clinical feature	*Score*	
Onset		
Loss of consciousness	One or none	0
Headache within 2 hours	Two or more	+21.9
Vomiting		
Neck stiffness		
Level of consciousness at 24 h		
	Alert	0
	Drowsy	+7.3
	Unconscious	+14.6
Plantar responses		
	Both flexor/single extensor	0
	Both extensor	+7.1
Diastolic BP at 24 h		
	BP mmHg	+(BP × 0.17)
History or atheroma markers		
Angina	None	0
Claudication	One or more	−3.7
Diabetes		
History of hypertension		
	Not present	0
	Present	−4.1
Previous TIA or stroke		
	None	0
	Previous event(s)	−6.7
Heart disease		
	None	0
	Aortic/mitral murmur	−4.3
	Cardiac failure	−4.3
	Cardiomyopathy	−4.3
	Atrial fibrillation	−4.3
	Cardiomegaly (X-ray)	−4.3
	Myocardial infarction within 6 months	−4.3
	Constant	*−12.6*

likelihood ratio shows that it is five times better than conventional clinical diagnosis in increasing the probability that a patient truly has a diagnosis of stroke due to cerebral haemorrhage.

This can be demonstrated by applying the likelihood ratios of conventional diagnosis and the Guy's Hospital score to the same pre-test odds. Assuming that the true frequency of haemorrhage is 0.20 (i.e. 20 per cent), this is equivalent to pre-test odds of 0.25.

Conventional clinical diagnosis (likelihood ratio 5.3):

$0.25 \times 5.3 = 1.325$ (posterior odds) $= 0.57$ probability
i.e. 57% predictive value.

Guy's Hospital score method (likelihood ratio 26):

$0.25 \times 26 = 6.5$ (posterior odds) $= 0.87$ probability
i.e. 87% predictive value.

The use of the Guy's Hospital score has been examined in two other series of patients, the Oxford Community Stroke Project patients and a series of patients from a London teaching hospital (Sandercock *et al.* 1985*b*). It was concluded that a cut-off of 4 would maximize the accuracy of the score (i.e. achieve the highest sensitivity and specificity). In practice, however, the task is to either rule out or rule in a diagnosis. To use a single cut-off point does not permit all the information contained in the score to be used. In general, highly abnormal values are more useful than borderline abnormalities in diagnosis. The data presented by Sandercock and colleagues is re-cast in Table 2.8 to show the diagnostic importance of different thresholds of the score.

It is evident from describing the score in this way that very high and very low scores have much greater diagnostic importance. The suggested threshold of four will achieve a predictive value of 45 per cent for cerebral haemorrhage in Oxford, whereas a threshold of 25 has a predictive value of 64 per cent and a threshold of less than −5 has a predictive value for cerebral infarction of about 98 per cent.

It is also of interest that the likelihood ratios for London teaching hospital patients are higher which is probably because they are much more clear-cut cases selected by primary care doctors, whereas the Oxford series included almost all cases from a defined population of patients in a community.

A clinical example. An example may clarify the use of the score.

Table 2.8 Use of the Guy's Hospital score among the Oxfordshire Community Stroke Project patients and London teaching hospital patients

Score Threshold	*Oxford patients*			*London teaching hospitals*		
	Haemorrhage			*Haemorrhage*		
	Present	*Absent*	*L.R.**	*Present*	*Absent*	*L.R.**
25+	9	5	8.0	43	2	50.9
14–24	13	9	6.4	15	4	8.9
4–13	12	27	2.0	20	38	1.2
−5–3	7	78	0.4	9	89	0.2
<−5	1	67	0.07	0	74	0
	42	186		87	206	

* *L.R.*, likelihood ratio.

A man of 73 presented to an Oxford hospital with sudden onset of left hemiplegia which was associated with loss of consciousness for at least two hours. He had a frontal headache when seen by a doctor 6 hours later. He was drowsy throughout the first day of hospital admission. He had a left extensor plantar, a diastolic phase (V) BP of 100 mmHg (phase IV, 110 mmHg) and was complaining of anginal chest pain when initially seen. He had a myocardial infarction 10 years earlier but no rhythm disturbance or heart failure. He had no previous neurological symptoms or past history of hypertension and his chest X-ray was normal. His Guy's Hospital score was:

$$21.9+7.3+0+(100\times 0.17)-3.7+0+0+0-12.6=29.9$$
$$\text{(or 31.6 if phase IV BP used).}$$

The prior odds of cerebral haemorrhage might be as low as 0.11 (i.e. 10 per cent probability). The Oxford likelihood ratios for this score is 8.0. This gives a posterior probability that this man has had a cerebral haemorrhage of 47 per cent. The same man admitted to a London Teaching Hospital would have a posterior Guy's Hospital probability of haemorrhage of 85 per cent. Such a high probability of haemorrhage is sufficient to rule out use of anti-coagulants or anti-platelet agents.

A decision about whether to use prophylactic subcutaneous heparin and aspirin could not be made without further investigation with computed tomography (CT) scanning as a cerebral haemorrhage appeared quite likely. If heparin and/or aspirin were given to such a patient, particularly in the early phase of the stroke, there is a danger that further haemorrhage will occur. The size of this risk is not known, and it can be argued that the trials of antiplatelet agents used for secondary prevention following stroke have not run into problems of exacerbating the stroke in patients with unsuspected cerebral haemorrhage. Several of these trials did not use CT scans to ensure that only patients with thrombo-embolic disease were treated, but entry into the trials was often late in the course of the stroke. It is unwise to assume on the strength of such trials that aspirin can be given to acute stroke patients without risk.

Lumbar puncture: an overlooked test?

A further advantage of likelihood ratios is that promising diagnostic methods are less likely to be overlooked. At present there is little enthusiasm for lumbar puncture to differentiate haemorrhagic from thrombotic stroke (Consensus Conference Report 1988). Yet the estimates of its likelihood ratio range from infinity (Harrison 1980) to 11 (Britton *et al.* 1983). It is possible that a combination of clinical scoring methods and lumbar puncture could produce predictive values of 97 to 99 per cent, which would mean that in only one case in 100 would a diagnosis of haemorrhage be wrong.

For example, if the pre-test odds of haemorrhagic stroke are 0.25 (i.e. 20 per cent, odds $= 0.2/1 - 0.2$), using a Guy's Hospital score (threshold of 14+) which has a likelihood ratio of 26:

$$0.25 \times 26 = \text{post-test odds} = 6.5.$$

The post-test odds may then be used as the pre-test odds for the application of another test, assuming independence between the tests. In this case lumbar puncture, which has a likelihood ratio of 11:

$$6.5 \times 11 = \text{post-test odds} = 71.5.$$

This is equivalent to a predictive value of:

$$71.5/(1 + 71.5) = 98.6\%.$$

If the probability of haemorrhagic stroke is lower than 20 per cent, say only 10 per cent, then use of the Guy's Hospital score and lumbar puncture gives a predictive value of 96.9 per cent. This strategy needs testing in an unselected series of patients to examine its true predictive value, as it is quite possible that the likelihood ratios of both the clinical score and lumbar puncture will not operate independently, that both methods will fail in a proportion of cases (inadequate information, bloody tap on lumbar puncture), and that their use may not be associated with such high predictive values in practice.

For some clinical decisions of relatively low risk (e.g. giving aspirin), the use of a clinical score and/or lumbar puncture may be good enough, but for others of higher risk (e.g. giving anticoagulants), this may not be accurate enough. Use of subcutaneous heparin for prophylaxis against deep vein thrombosis and pulmonary emboli is a particularly difficult case. Small trials have been conducted without CT scanning to exclude cerebral haemorrhages and iatrogenic bleeding problems have not been reported. The obvious solution is to conduct a CT scan in any patient for whom subcutaneous heparin is to be used, and to avoid heparin where a haemorrhagic lesion is found on CT scan. An alternative approach is to weigh the risks and benefits of subcutaneous heparin using a decision tree (see Chapter 4). For epidemiological purposes such as describing trends or differences in occurrence between places, or times, or characteristics of individuals (e.g. smoking, blood pressure, etc.) the level of diagnostic accuracy achieved by clinical scoring and/or lumbar puncture is more than adequate.

Lacunar stroke

The clinical diagnosis of lacunar stroke can be made if a patient presents with a pure motor stroke, a pure sensory stroke, ataxic hemiparesis, and sensori-motor stroke. The relationship between these clinical presentations and finding an appropriate 'lacuna' or small deep infarct on CT scanning is variable. The sensitivity and specificity of these lacunar presentations can be tested by comparison with CT scan findings. The sensitivity ranges from less than 35 per cent to 69 per cent with a small deep infarct, and the false-positive rate from 7 per cent to 14 per cent, who turned out to have a cerebral haemorrhage (Bamford and Warlow 1988). This gives a likelihood ratio of 10 at best, which suggests that the syndrome can be detected by clinicians with reasonable accuracy. However, the importance of making the diagnosis is not yet clear (Weisberg 1988).

Summary

1. The accuracy with which doctors distinguish vascular strokes (i.e. infarcts, emboli, haemorrhages) from other non-vascular pathology ranges from a sensitivity of 67 to 100 per cent, and a specificity of 22 to 91 per cent. Variation is due to the clinical skill of the doctor, the age range of patients studied, and the clinical setting from which the series of patients were collected (i.e. hospital, specialist stroke unit).

2. Up to 13 per cent of patients thought initially to have had a stroke turn out to have some other pathology. The commonest causes of diagnostic error are epilepsy, including Todd's paresis, delirium, and loss of consciousness (drugs, alcohol, metabolic, intercurrent illness, orthostatic syncope), mass lesions (subdural haematomas, tumours), depression, and dementia syndromes.

3. Clinical methods (scoring and lumbar puncture) may be used to distinguish haemorrhagic from thrombo-embolic stroke with sufficient accuracy (predictive value up to 99 per cent) for epidemiological purposes, and probably for use of anti-platelet agents in secondary prevention for patients with thrombo-embolic stroke. Further work is needed to define the accuracy of this approach. Clinical methods are unlikely to be accurate enough to help us decide on the use of anticoagulants in stroke patients.

4. The clinical diagnosis of lacunar stroke is reasonably accurate, but the value of making this diagnosis is not clear.

3 Clinical disagreement

Variation in eliciting history and signs

Whenever two or more doctors are asked to assess the same patient it is unlikely that they will agree completely on their clinical findings. This phenomenon is well recognized in several fields of medicine, ranging from taking a history (Cochrane *et al.* 1951), examination of the pedal pulses (Meade *et al.* 1968), chest examination (Spiteri *et al.* 1988), to interpretation of exercise electrocardiograms (Blackburn *et al.* 1968). It is not surprising, therefore, that in the assessment of stroke patients agreement is not absolute. Information on which doctors disagree can be considered in terms of its importance to diagnosis, management, and prognosis. If the information is crucial, every effort must be made to reduce disagreements; if the information is of little value, there is no point in wasting time collecting it, much less trying to improve its reliability. For example, if two clinicians disagree on the presence of a carotid bruit the patient may or may not be exposed to the risk of angiograms (or denied the benefits of investigation and treatment) depending on one's point of view. Disagreements on factors that determine rehabilitation potential (e.g. mental state, severity of stroke, pre-stroke ability) may lead to patients being denied access to therapy and discharged to nursing homes inappropriately or before their full potential has been achieved.

In one study (Garraway *et al.* 1976), four consultants examined 12 patients looking for seven impairments that might be caused by an acute stroke. The overall agreement between the four doctors was only 34 (41 per cent) out of a total of 84 (i.e. 12×7) possible agreements. Agreements for assessment of mental function, proprioception, posture, and motor function were low, whereas spatial neglect, comprehension and expression showed reasonable agreement.

Disagreements are also found in taking a history, as demonstrated by an Italian study (Tomasello *et al.* 1982), where the question of observer variation was important as a multi-centre study was being undertaken. Agreement between eight examiners of 55 patients who had suffered recurrent transient ischaemic attacks or minor strokes was measured using an 'index of agreement' (the ratio of the number of subjects with agreement in responses to the total number of patients). Using this index, around 50 per cent agreement was found for both the frequency and number of transient ischaemic attacks. Agreement on neurological symptoms was higher, with 66 per cent agreement on the presence of visual, sensory or speech impairments and higher agreement (76 per cent) on motor impairments. The examiners did better on neurological signs with high agreement for visual field defects (92 per cent), but agreement on cerebellar signs (37.5 per cent), sensory signs (25 per cent), and plantar responses (21 per cent) were all low.

It is perhaps even more surprising that agreement was low as a standardized data record was used by all examiners. The authors concluded that disagreements may have been due to differences in the interests of the examiners, the motivation of the patients, imperfect recall of short-lived symptoms, and differences in dialect, education, and social status between examiners and patients.

Chance levels of agreement

The level of agreement in this Italian study was overestimated by the index of agreement used. The index used is affected by the frequency of a particular abnormality, for example, if a sign is rare (e.g. cranial bruit) or very common (e.g. motor weakness), then even if there is little agreement between examiners, a high level of chance agreement will be found. For example, assuming that Observer 1 thinks that 10 per cent of stroke patients have sensory impairments and 90 per cent do not, and Observer 2 thinks that the proportions are 20 per cent and 80 per cent respectively, then the probability that both observers will agree on the *absence* of sensory impairment, without even examining the patient is:

$$0.90 \times 0.80 = 0.72, \text{ i.e. } 72\%$$

This is because the rules of probability require independent probabilities to be multiplied together to produce the probability of two events occurring. In this case the events are Observers 1 and 2 agreeing on the absence of a sign. The probability that both observers will agree on the *presence* of sensory impairment, again without examining the patient is:

$$0.10 \times 0.20 = 0.02, \text{ i.e. } 2\%$$

This adds up to an overall agreement of 74 per cent, as shown in Table 3.1.

The chance association between their findings (the body of Table 3.1) is obtained in the same way as calculating the expected values for a chi-square (χ^2) 2×2 table. The product of each row and column total is divided by the grand total (e.g. $(90 \times 80)/100 = 72$). The crude percentage agreement looks quite acceptable, 74 per cent, but this 'agreement' was, of course, produced entirely by using expected chance levels of association. Note also that this chance level of agreement is higher than many of the levels of agreement reported in the Italian study! In other words, many of the observed agreements could easily have been due to chance rather than any consistency between examiners.

With more common or rarer findings (e.g. weakness or neck rigidity), the percentage crude agreement becomes an even less good estimate of the true level of agreement as shown in Table 3.2. This level of agreement looks very impressive when reported as an

Table 3.1 Chance association in agreement between two observers where Observer 1 decides the prevalence of abnormality is 10% and Observer 2 uses a prevalence of 20% abnormality

Observer 2	*Observer 1*		
	No sensory impairment	*Sensory impairment*	
No sensory impairment	72	8	80
Sensory impairment	18	2	20
	90	10	100

Crude percentage agreement 72 + 2/100 = 74%.

Table 3.2 Chance agreement between two observers when Observer 1 thinks that 1% of patients have neck rigidity and Observer 2 thinks that 2% have the sign

Observer 2	*Observer 1*		
	Neck rigidity	*No neck rigidity*	
Neck rigidity	0.02	1.98	2.00
No neck rigidity	0.98	97.02	98.00
	1.00	99.00	100.00

Crude percentage chance agreement (97.02 + 0.02)/100 = 97%.

observed level of agreement, but once again it is entirely the result of chance.

Adjusting for chance agreement

The Cohen's kappa statistic (Cohen 1960) allows for this chance variation by subtracting the chance agreement from the observed agreement, and expressing this chance-adjusted agreement as a proportion of the potential real agreement possible (i.e. 100 per cent minus the chance agreement), i.e.

$$\text{kappa} = \kappa = (P_O - P_C)/(1 - P_C)$$

where P_O is the observed proportion of agreement and P_C is the expected chance proportion of agreement. It is usual to express these proportions as numbers between 0 and 1 rather than as percentages. Consequently kappa will range from +1 for complete agreement to −1 for complete disagreement, and a value of zero will indicate only chance agreement. The chi-square statistic can be used to give a significance level to the kappa value.

The observed agreement with this hypothetical data is: (20 + 60)/100 = 80% or 0.80, which seems quite acceptable, and the chi-square value is 28.22 which suggest that it was highly unlikely to have arisen by chance. The numbers in brackets are the expected or chance values which give a chance agreement of:

$$(10.9 + 44.9)/100 = 55.8\% \text{ or } 0.558.$$

Table 3.3 Observed and chance agreement between two observers on a prior history of stroke, assumed to be present in 33%. Numbers in brackets are those expected by chance

Observer 2	*Observer 1*		
	Past history	*No past history*	
Past history	20 (10.9)	7 (22.1)	33
No past history	13 (22.1)	60 (44.9)	67
	33	67	100

Observed agreement = 80%; chance agreement = 55.8%.

The kappa statistic is:

$$\kappa = (0.80 - 0.558)/(1 - 0.558) = 0.55$$

which indicates only moderate agreement once the effects of chance have been taken into account. Levels over 0.75 are usually taken to indicate excellent agreement (Landis and Koch 1977). In this example, to exceed this kappa value, crude percentage agreement would have to be at least 90 per cent.

An American study measured the agreement between six neurologists who examined 17 stroke patients over the course of three days, using a balanced design in which each patient was seen by four of the doctors (Shinar *et al.* 1985). As each patient was seen four times, a total of 68 possible agreements were available for each piece of information. Answers to apparently straightforward questions were subject to disagreement. The history of a previous stroke was agreed upon on 45 (66 per cent) of the 68 occasions, with similar levels of agreement for presence of headache at onset, and past history of a transient ischaemic attack. Perfect agreement by all four doctors was achieved much less often: past history of stroke—35 per cent; headache at onset—41 per cent; transient ischaemic attack in the past—29 per cent. These authors also used the kappa statistic to adjust for the level of chance agreement. Surprisingly, only two items of history achieved good agreement: alcohol ingestion within 24 hours of stroke (kappa = 0.65), and time of last meal (kappa = 0.46). Other important information such as level of consciousness, seizure at onset, headache, vomiting, and the course of the illness over the first 24 hours only achieved modest agreement (kappa values from 0.32 to 0.39). Presence of a focal deficit at onset, previous transient ischaemic attack, deficit present on waking, and use of anti-coagulants or anti-platelet agents all showed levels of only chance agreement with kappa values from 0.15 to 0.08.

The crude percentage agreements of neurological signs were shown to be quite misleading and no better than history-taking. Kappa values showed excellent agreement for the following: swallowing; deviation of eyes; articulation and speech impairment; side of hemiplegia. Only chance levels of agreement were found for the following: tongue weakness; depressed mood; neck stiffness; cervical bruits; and pure motor syndrome.

Observer variation in the type of stroke (i.e. haemorrhagic, embolic, lacunar, thrombotic) has also been studied (Gross *et al.* 1986). Using the same study design and patients as referred to above, each of the four doctors seeing the 17 patients was asked to give a provisional diagnosis after taking a history and examining the patient. Complete agreement on diagnosis was achieved for only seven (41 per cent, kappa 0.38) of the 17 when the categories of infarction were combined into a single group, otherwise there was no case in which each neurologist agreed on the particular diagnosis. Further diagnostic work-up, which included CT scans for every patient, improved agreement: 10 (59 per cent) perfect agreements (kappa 0.69) when infarction was a single category, and 6 (35 per cent) perfect agreements (kappa 0.61) when sub-categories of infarction were considered.

Improving clinical agreement

Definition, standardization, and explanation

We must therefore accept that disagreement exists and that it is sufficiently undesirable that something should be done about it. Only one study has attempted to measure the impact of strategies to improve agreement (Garraway *et al.* 1976). The method used was to define categories more closely, and to standardize the method of examination. This led to improvements in the agreement on motor function, spatial neglect, proprioception, comprehension/expression, and mental function. Postural function (i.e. balance and posture) remained difficult to agree on. Despite improvements, side of hemiplegia was inaccurately recorded on six out of 12 patients by one or more of the examining doctors! This was probably the result of using 'CVA' as a diagnostic label with inevitable confusion between the side of hemisphere damage and the side of the hemiplegia. As well as defining categories more carefully and standardization of examination techniques, doctors need to be more careful about the terms used to describe strokes.

Further explanation and discussion with the doctors, increased standardization of terms and recording methods led to further improvements in agreement. With considerable effort it was possible to improve overall agreements from 41 to 68 per cent of all items measured and to reduce between observer differences in function scores to a quarter of the differences observed before training. This study also demonstrated that not only do doctors disagree with each other, they are not particularly consistent from one week to the next in their own opinions. Inconsistency ranged from 17 to 31 per cent of all items assessed, with the biggest differences in mental function, proprioception, and motor function.

This study was undertaken because several different doctors were to assess patients in a trial of the effects of a stroke unit. Agreement between doctors was essential to ensure comparability between those assessed in the stroke unit and those managed on medical wards. Despite the training it is quite possible that with time, doctors would drift back to their usual practice and disagreements would recur. In long-term studies it is usually necessary to ensure that observers have regular training sessions to ensure standards of agreement are maintained. In routine clinical practice this should be an integral part of continuing education.

Information value

Defining the information that is essential for diagnosis, management, and prognosis is a useful starting point. There is little point in refining the techniques of measurement for information of little practical value. Table 3.4 attempts to classify information about stroke patients according to its potential value in each of these three areas. Only side of weakness, speech impairment, orientation, swallowing, and gaze paresis have reasonable levels of clinical agreement (Shinar *et al.* 1985).

Perceptual impairment requires training to improve agreement,

Table 3.4 A classification of information for its use in diagnosis, management, and prognosis, together with the level of clinical agreement

Diagnosis	*Management*	*Prognosis*
Side of weakness[a]	Side of weakness[a]	
Speech impairment[a]	Speech impairment[a]	Speech impairment[a]
Previous stroke	Swallowing[a]	Swallowing[a]
Mode of onset	Perceptual loss[b]	Perceptual loss[b]
Stroke risk factors	Orientation[b]	Orientation[b]
Headache	Degree of weakness	Gaze paresis[a]
Vomiting	Conscious level	Conscious level
Photophobia	Mood	Mood
Neck stiffness	Balance/gait	Balance/gait
	Continence[c]	Continence[c]
	Visual field loss	Visual field loss
	Pre-stroke ability[c]	Pre-stroke ability[c]
	Type of stroke	Type of stroke

[a] Good clinical agreement.
[b] Good agreement after training.
[c] Agreement level not known.
All others show only poor to chance levels of agreement.

and some important information such as continence of urine, pre-stroke ability, presence of stroke risk factors (e.g. high blood pressure, diabetes, smoking) has not been assessed for clinical agreement. All the other information listed has been shown to have low levels of clinical agreement.

The next step to improve agreement is to consider the reasons for disagreement and to decide what (if anything) can be done about them. The McMaster group (Sackett *et al.* 1985) have classified sources of variation as due to the examiner, the examined and the examination.

The examiner

Fatigue is likely to be a major cause of disagreement: it has been shown that tired doctors make more mistakes when interpreting ECGs (Friedman *et al.* 1971). Traditionally the neurological part of the clinical examination is left until last and by this time, particularly if the patient is deaf or delirious, a reliable examination is unlikely. Some doctors record a diagnosis of 'Right CVA' when they mean that the patient has a left hemiplegia (or right hemisphere damage). This shorthand leads to much confusion because it is not clear whether the 'right' refers to the brain or the body. It is better to record observations and not inferences from observations. Elderly patients suffer strokes most frequently, and are not easy to examine. Consequently, doctors can easily fail to record information that is essential to diagnosis, management or prognosis because of a technically poor examination. This may be because of ignorance (several medical schools in the United Kingdom still do not have academic departments of geriatric medicine to teach such skills), disinterest or an assumption that having diagnosed a stroke not much can (or should) be done for the patient.

The examined

Dysphasia, cognitive impairments, depressed conscious level, and associated problems will all make history-taking and physical signs more prone to variability, especially in the acute phase. As symptoms and signs improve (or deteriorate) quite rapidly in the early phase, and extra items of information are discovered (from helpful relatives, neighbours, family doctors, etc.), it is sensible to consider the initial examination as just the beginning of the data collection and interpretation process.

The examination

The hospital ward or emergency room environment is not usually conducive to testing higher cognitive function or enquiring about sensitive issues such as urinary continence, because of noise and the urge to get to the next patient. This may also lead to a poor doctor-patient interaction, especially if a patient's hearing aid, spectacles, and false teeth are not used appropriately and if the patient is lying uncomfortably on an examination trolley. The situation is not helped if the doctor is simultaneously interrogating the patient, answering a telephone call, and trying to find a bed for the patient.

Solutions

Some solutions are obvious but not often implemented. Doctors should do an examination appropriate to the task in hand. In the emergency room the aim is to assess the urgency of the clinical condition of the patient and the need for admission. The admitting physician's job is to ensure that the diagnosis of a vascular stroke is reasonably likely, that other causes of neurological impairment (e.g. hypoglycaemia, meningitis, mass lesions, etc.) have been excluded and that information for immediate management has been obtained (e.g. swallowing, medication, need for pressure sore prevention). The subsequent tasks are to collect and interpret information to aid subsequent management and give a prognosis. This needs to be done using multiple sources (e.g. the patient, ward staff, old records, home support services, friends, etc.), and may require a series of small focused examinations of the patient in a quiet environment. These tasks are easy to neglect.

Sackett and colleagues (1985) recommend repeating key findings, and asking colleagues to examine the patient unguided by prior knowledge of the findings, which is part of the tradition of bedside teaching. It does, of course, imply that doctors have sufficient knowledge to elicit signs in the first place. Sackett suggests that serious faults in medical education exist when it is possible for doctors to reach advanced stages of training without ever having their technique of interviewing or examining watched and criticized by another colleague or teacher. Certainly, the standard examination of stroke patients in the United Kingdom might lead one to believe that patients do not have any higher cortical function, apart from the motor cortex, and comprise merely of cranial nerves (usually reported as intact, although smell is seldom, if ever, tested), and spinal reflex arcs.

Another approach to improve agreement is to replace the traditional blank page upon which doctors write their findings with a more systematic preprinted record of essential information to be collected. Routine use of mental test scores (mainly concerned with memory and orientation) is common in geriatric medical practice, and this approach should be extended to include standardized assessments of other useful information, such as mood, perceptual impairment, and pre-stroke ability.

Summary

1. Disagreement in clinical findings between even well-trained clinicians is common.

2. The usual methods of reporting ageement as a crude percentage of observed to total possible agreements does not allow for chance association, and tends to overestimate the degree of agreement. Kappa values are chance-adjusted and give a more reliable measure of agreement.

3. Agreement about historical information (such as history of a previous stroke, use of anti-platelet drugs), and physical signs (carotid bruits, neck stiffness, side of stroke) is poor and often no better than chance agreement.

4. It is necessary to define which information is necessary for diagnosis, management, and prognosis and to attempt to improve the reliability of the collection of this information. Other information of questionable reliability and value should be discarded.

5. Improved standardization of examination methods, record keeping, and appropriate task-orientated examination, together with more direct observation of clinical technique may lead to improved clinical agreement.

4 Investigation

Computed tomographic (CT) scanning

Who needs a CT scan?

The question of which patients merit a CT scan does not arise for many stroke patients. Hospital admission for patients sustaining a stroke in the UK varies from around half to three-quarters (Oxfordshire Community Stroke Project 1983; Barer *et al.* 1984) admitted. It is certainly possible to arrange a CT scan for those patients remaining at home. In the Oxford study (where an attempt to CT scan all patients was made) a creditable 80 per cent of all stroke patients were scanned. However, there were delays, with only 62 per cent of both hospital and community patients getting a scan within three weeks of onset of the stroke. After this time it is quite possible that small haemorrhages will have resolved (Dennis *et al.* 1987) and will be no longer visible on CT scan films.

The Oxford group have defined patients who require a CT scan as those who have an atypical clinical course; are young (although age is not defined); those in whom treatment with antiplatelet or anticoagulant drugs might be used; and those where there is diagnostic doubt (Sandercock *et al.* 1985*a*; Warlow 1987). While these criteria seem sensible it is difficult to find evidence to support them.

Atypical clinical course. Evidence that an atypical, stuttering, or prolonged onset of symptoms and signs is relatively more common among patients with a nonvascular cause for their neurological impairment is equivocal (Weisberg and Nice 1977; Allen 1983; Sandercock *et al.* 1985*a*). In those studies that found such an association, the predictive value of this information is quite low (see Chapter 2 on diagnosis). If a CT scan was done for every patient with an atypical onset of stroke, from 1.3 per cent (Sandercock *et al.* 1985*a*) to 14 per cent (Allen 1983) of patients would turn out to have a nonvascular lesion. The majority would have a stroke, and around four-fifths (Sandercock *et al.* 1985*a*) to one-half

(Allen 1983) of nonvascular lesions would be missed because they did not present with an unusual onset.

Younger patients. The rationale for an age criterion is that rare causes of stroke (e.g. arterio-venous malformations, aneurysms, angiomas) are more frequent and are more often treatable. The difficulty is in deciding on an age threshold. Some nonvascular lesions become *more* common with age and are just as treatable as in younger patients—in particular subdural haematomas and meningiomas. Up to the age of 75 it is likely that many neurosurgeons will consider evacuating a subdural haematoma. After this age, the overall condition of the patient may determine the feasibility and likely prognosis of surgery. If an age criterion is to be used then it seems illogical to set it much below 75 years of age if the purpose is to detect clinically unrecognized but surgically treatable pathology.

Use of anti-platelet agents or anti-coagulants. Anti-platelet agents are of established benefit in preventing fatal and non-fatal vascular events among patients with mild strokes and TIAs (Anti-platelet Trialists Collaboration 1988). It is likely that their use will be expanded to include all stroke survivors. This indication for CT scanning would lead to a dramatic increase in its use and would require a massive investment in scanning facilities in the United Kingdom. Anti-coagulants are of no proven benefit to patients after stroke (see Chapter 8 on reducing the risks of recurrent stroke), but if they are required for thrombo-embolic disease such as pulmonary embolus or mitral stenosis with atrial fibrillation, then it is sensible to ensure that the patient is not put at risk of bleeding into a haemorrhagic infarct or of worsening a cerebral haemorrhage.

The use of subcutaneous heparin for prophylaxis against deep vein thrombosis and pulmonary emboli is problematic. Treatment must be started early as deep vein thromboses are most likely in the first few days, but it may take several days to organize a CT scan, particularly if the purpose is to exclude a cerebral haemorrhage. The small trial of sub-cutaneous heparin (McCarthy and Turner 1986) did not use CT scanning to exclude haemorrhagic lesions, but treated all stroke patients. Although no adverse effects of treatment were found, the trial was too small to give reliable estimates of the likely risks of treatment among patients with cerebral haemorrhage or haemorrhagic infarction. Further studies of sub-cutaneous heparin should attempt to examine the risks and relative benefits of treatment for such patients.

Diagnostic doubt. A clinical diagnosis of vascular stroke can never be absolutely certain. Doctors differ in the degree of uncertainty that they can tolerate and if a CT scan is done merely to check that a highly probably diagnosis is true, then this is wasteful of resources. It is quite possible that time is the most useful clinical tool for distinguishing strokes from nonvascular disease, watching the course of the patient's illness over a few days to two weeks. Unfortunately, no systematic studies of this strategy have been carried out so it is not yet possible to measure its sensitivity and specificity in diagnosing nonvascular problems. It would be sensible to monitor not just neurological signs, but also functional ability (sitting balance, transfers, walking, feeding, dressing, etc.), and cognitive state (using the Mini-mental State Examination, for example, Folstein *et al.* 1975). Patients with a deteriorating or static course or with disproportionate impairment of consciousness might be the right ones to investigate with CT scanning. Another approach is to ask the question 'what caused this stroke?'. It is possible that if the patient has risk factors for stroke (other than age) then it is less necessary to consider nonvascular pathology. At present there is no clear answer whether either of these approaches is useful.

Accuracy of CT scans

The accuracy of a CT scan in diagnosing a stroke is given by its sensitivity and specificity, but a difficulty arises because, apart from an autopsy, the only suitable standard for comparison, cerebral angiography, is risky. However, if a clinician diagnoses a stroke on history and examination, but nothing is seen on the CT scan, an estimate of the sensitivity (or false-negative rate) can be made. In practice, false-negative scans are common—around 20–40 per cent of all scans (Wade *et al.* 1985*b*), and there is a tendency to interpret them as representing cerebral infarcts (Oxfordshire Community Stroke Project 1983).

It is less likely that patients thought clinically not to have a stroke will be CT scanned, so reliable estimates of the specificity (or false-positive rate) are difficult to obtain. Comparison with autopsy diagnosis has been tried (Toghi *et al.* 1981), but patients undergoing both a CT scan and an autopsy are hardly typical of most patients suffering a stroke.

The major determinant of whether the CT scan will identify a stroke is the size of the lesion. Small lesions are more often missed, leading to the low observed sensitivity, and it is easy to over-interpret a CT scan leading to a false-positive diagnosis of stroke when nothing is found at autopsy (Toghi *et al.* 1981). Timing of the CT scan is critical, and unless the CT scan and autopsy are performed within a few days of each other, it is quite possible that a small CT lesion will have resolved, or be missed quite easily at autopsy, meaning that the autopsy is perhaps not as accurate as CT scanning in some cases.

Variations in interpretation

Variation in the interpretation of CT scans has been reported among patients with brain tumours (Swets *et al.* 1979) and stroke (Shinar *et al.* 1987). Although CT scans are often considered to be the 'gold standard' against which clinical and other investigations should be compared, it is worth remembering that interpretation of an image is subjective and consequently liable to observer variation. Variation should be less marked for examination of CT scans than for clinical history and examination (see Chapter 3 on clinical disagreement) because two major sources of variation do not exist—the patients cannot vary, neither can the way in which the examination is performed.

When six neurologists were asked to report the CT scans of 17 patients, excellent agreement was achieved when the categories were grouped as 'normal', 'haemorrhage', 'infarct', and 'other'; all six agreed on 13 out of 17 scans, and five out of six neurologists agreed on three of the remaining four patients, with a kappa coefficient of 0.90, which indicates a very high level of agreement. However, on two CT scans which five and four of the six neurologists declared normal, one reported a deep, large infarct and two found deep, small infarcts respectively. Although it might be thought that haemorrhages and infarcts would not be confused, one neurologist reported both an infarct and a haemorrhage, and aneurysms and arteriovenous malformations were detected on several occasions in the presence of both haemorrhage and infarcts.

When the neurologists were asked to describe the location of lesions, perhaps surprisingly they found on average two lesions per CT scan, which made arriving at an agreement on location of lesion rather complicated. They could distinguish reasonably well whether a lesion was superficial, deep, in the cerebellum or extracerebral space but more particular locations, such as thalamus, operculum, and insula were not agreed upon at all well. The side of the main lesion, lesion density, mass effect, oedema, and lesion size were subject to moderate to poor agreement (kappa 0.65 to 0.34) (Shinar *et al.* 1987).

These neurologists tended to over-interpret the CT scans and this led to a glut of diagnoses, which in some cases might have resulted in more invasive investigations. It is clearly unwise to expect much agreement on the precise location of lesions, their size, and their effects (i.e. oedema, mass effect). The implication of this is that attempts to use such information for correlation with clinical presentation, symptoms, signs, and progress requires that either a single observer is used (and there is no published information on within-observer variation), or that more standardized criteria are used when reporting CT scans.

The value of CT scanning

The value of any investigation can be assessed in three ways: the proportion of altered diagnoses; the proportion of patients whose management is changed; and finally the number of lives saved or disability prevented. As a major emphasis in medicine is the art of diagnosis, it is easy to over-value the importance of altered diagnoses. CT scanning makes only a small contribution to diagnosis of stroke from other conditions that mimic it. Its main use is in characterizing mass lesions such as subdural haematoma, primary and secondary neoplasms, and abscesses.

Altered diagnoses

The Oxfordshire Community Stroke Project (Sandercock *et al.* 1985*a*) has provided some of the best data on the diagnostic changes produced by a policy of universal CT scanning of stroke patients. Only patients with a first stroke were included in this study, and 89 per cent were seen by a neurologist early in the course of the illness. Only five (1.5 per cent) out of 325 patients turned out to have unsuspected nonvascular pathology. In two patients this was a subdural haematoma, but only one was treated surgically and the other was not treated because of her age (86 years) and general condition. Two patients with gliomas both died.

The amount of unsuspected nonvascular pathology found may, in part, reflect the clinical skills of doctors and the source of patients studied. In the Oxford study, primary care doctors referred 736 patients as suitable for the study, of whom only 325 (44 per cent) were considered to have suffered a first stroke by the neurologist, who was able to pick out clinically 16 of the 21 patients with space-occupying lesions. Allen's series of patients (1983) included nine (5 per cent) out of 174 found to have nonvascular pathology. An early American series (Weisberg and Nice 1977) found 18 (20 per cent) out of 90 patients had tumours or subdural haematomas. Older patients might be expected to have a higher risk of nonvascular pathology, but among 79 patients aged 65 to 97 years, admitted to hospital, only one (1 per cent) astrocytoma was detected (O'Brien *et al.* 1987). It is clear that clinical history-taking and examination is of great value in distinguishing strokes from nonvascular pathology.

Altered management

Clinicians might value knowing the 'true' diagnosis, or ruling out a particular diagnosis. The value of this increased certainty should be measured in terms of its impact on changes in management. For example, if a CT scan shows a massive cerebral infarct in a patient with impaired consciousness then further investigations to establish the cause of unconsciousness will not be necessary and intensive treatment, such as ventilation, might not be started. The effects on management can be considered under several headings: anti-platelet agents; anti-coagulants; surgery; and palliative treatments (e.g. dexamethasone, radiotherapy, hospice care).

Anti-platelet agents. In the Oxford study 11 (3 per cent) of 325 patients were on aspirin at the time of their stroke. One patient had had a cerebral haemorrhage and aspirin was therefore stopped, and seven had no evidence of haemorrhage and treatment was continued. The remaining three were not scanned and it is not clear what happened to their treatment. Presumably most of the 119 (37 per cent) patients with CT scan-proven cerebral infarcts would be eligible for treatment with aspirin (provided they survived the acute phase of their stroke and had no contraindication to its use) and could be started on it safely. The 106 (33 per cent) patients with a CT scan that showed no lesion or only atrophy may be classified as thrombo-embolic strokes as the Oxford group did, but this prejudges the issue. It is quite possible that they may have suffered small haemorrhages which had resolved by the time a CT scan was carried out. The safety of giving aspirin to such patients must remain in doubt.

Anti-coagulants. Some clinicians use anti-coagulants for patients who have suffered a stroke and have atrial fibrillation. There is no evidence to support this practice but a CT scan showing no evidence of cerebral haemorrhage might make it slightly safer. The Oxford study found 46 (14 per cent) patients had atrial fibrillation, two had cerebral haemorrhages, and one a haemorrhagic infarct, 11 were not investigated, and a further three patients had haemorrhagic lesions found at autopsy. CT scanning thus showed that anti-coagulant treatment was potentially unsafe in three to 14 patients.

Surgery. Evacuation of a cerebellar haematoma can be considered provided an early diagnosis is made. The Oxford study detected only one patient with a cerebellar haematoma during life, out of five that occurred in their series. This patient was not offered surgery.

Although of no proven benefit carotid endarterectomy (see Chapter 8 on reducing the risk of recurrent stroke) might be offered to patients. The Oxford study found 19 (6 per cent) patients potentially eligible for this operation. CT scanning showed that two of them had had cerebral haemorrhages and they were not therefore investigated as a prelude to surgery.

Evacuation of subdural haematomas and excision of accessible meningiomas are of benefit to some patients. Although the Oxford study detected two patients with subdural haematomas only one was operated on with a successful outcome. The results of surgery for subdural haematoma are probably age-dependent with a trend for 'conservative' management to be given to patients in their eighties, thus reducing the value of making this diagnosis, especially in very old, frail patients.

Palliative treatment. Only two (0.6 per cent) patients with unsuspected primary brain tumours were discovered in the Oxford study. The CT scan led to a change in their management in that they were given dexamethasone, and presumably attempts at rehabilitation were stopped. Both died.

Lives saved and disability prevented

On this measure of the value of CT scanning, the following might be included: the patient with a successfully treated subdural haematoma; the three patients with atrial fibrillation and cerebral haemorrhage who might have died or got worse if they had been anti-coagulated; the two patients with cerebral haemorrhage who might have had a risky angiogram to define their suitability for carotid endarterectomy. It is worth noting that neither anti-coagulation or endarterectomy are of proven value, thus are not treatments that would even be considered by many UK clinicians. So between one and six (0.3–1.8 per cent) patients out of 325 considered in the Oxford study definitely benefited from CT scanning in terms of lives saved or disability prevented.

Other investigations

Investigation of stroke patients should be aimed at detecting those patients with nonvascular pathology. The Oxfordshire community stroke project reported that only 4% of 244 patients with an apparent first stroke turned out to have non-atheromatous, non-embolic causes for their symptoms and signs (Sandercock *et al.* 1989). A further 105 had no discernible cause for their stroke, but the majority of patients had risk factors: hypertension (52 per cent); coexisting ischaemic heart disease (38 per cent); diabetes (10 per cent); and a past history of transient ischaemic attack (14 per cent). The authors considered that a full blood count, ESR, blood glucose, urea and electrolytes, syphilis serology, chest X-ray and ECG should be sufficient to identify most patients with nonvascular pathology. The patients in this series had all been seen by a neurologist early in the course of their stroke, and a large number of patients thought to have had a stroke by their family doctor were excluded from further consideration by the study neurologists. Few would wish to quibble with the investigations suggested by Sandercock and colleagues, but it is likely that a minority of patients in the

United Kingdom will get these tests done, particularly those managed at home.

Clinical decision tree analysis

An alternative approach to deciding how to use an investigation is to construct a clinical decision tree. The utility of a test depends on its accuracy (i.e. sensitivity and specificity), the frequency of outcomes of interest, and also on the value placed on the information obtained. Figure 4.1 shows a simple decision tree for use of a CT scan to detect nonvascular pathology. As CT scanning is currently the best investigation for detection of nonvascular pathology the sensitivity and sensitivity can both be assumed to be

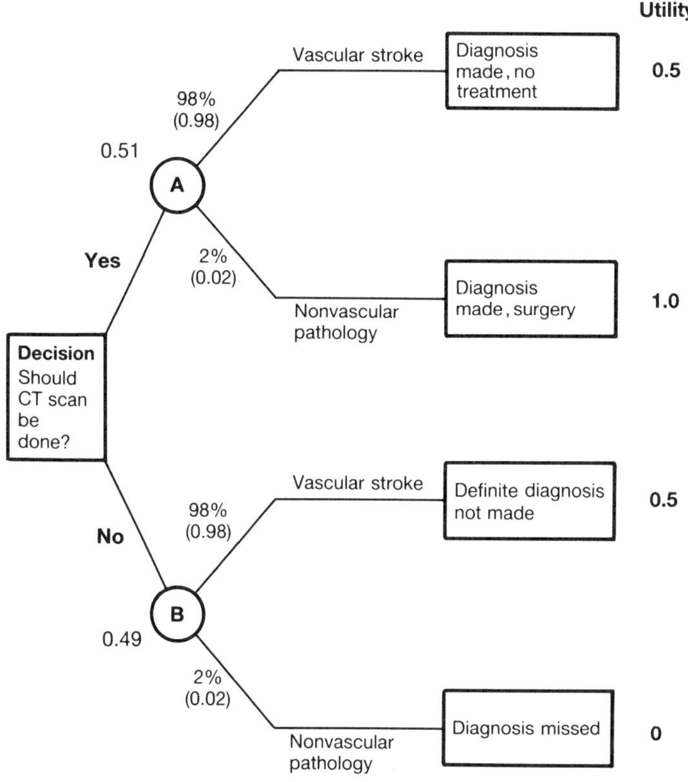

Fig. 4.1 Decision tree: CT scanning to diagnose nonvascular pathology.

100 per cent. At circle A, there is a 98 per cent probability that a stroke will be found and an approximately 2 per cent chance that nonvascular pathology will be found. Both arms are labelled with the probabilities. Similarly at circle B, the same probabilities will occur. The clinician will arrive at four possible outcomes which will be of different value:

1. A diagnosis of stroke made, but no available treatment.
2. A diagnosis of subdural haematoma, meningioma, etc., where surgical treatment may be of great benefit.
3. No definite diagnosis made, but no available treatment anyway.
4. A diagnosis of nonvascular pathology missed, which might have been surgically treatable.

Each outcome of investigation with CT scanning has a different value; but what value? Readers might care to rank the outcomes from worst to best in an effort to decide on their own values. In general to miss a potentially treatable diagnosis is bad, and in the example shown has been given a score (or utility) of zero. The best outcome might be to make a diagnosis where there is at least a possibility of surgery leading to complete recovery; this has been given a value of 1.0. The other two outcomes seem to have little to choose between them and have both been given a utility of 0.5. Note that utilities, like probabilities take values from 0 to 1. Readers may disagree with the values given and can try the effect of substituting different values for the utility of each outcome.

The next step in using the decision tree is to work backwards from the utility of a particular outcome, calculating how likely it is to occur. As 98 per cent (or 0.98) of CT scans will demonstrate a stroke of utility 0.5, the overall utility of this branch of the tree is 0.98×0.5 (i.e. 0.49). To this must be added the utility of the lower branch of the tree; the extremely valuable (utility = 1), but rather rare (0.02) diagnosis of nonvascular pathology which gives an extra utility of 0.02×1 (i.e. 0.02) to add to the upper branch utility (i.c. 0.51). This is the utility (or value) measured in the arbitrary units of value used in the example.

The decision not to do a CT scan gives a utility of 0.49, because the missed diagnosis of nonvascular pathology is such a disaster that it contributes nothing to the utility of this decision. The overall picture is neither for nor against doing a CT scan on every stroke patient, if the main purpose is to diagnose and treat nonvascular pathology. Indeed, if a branch is included for the later diagnosis of some nonvascular pathology which becomes clinically obvious, then the utility of not doing a CT scan will clearly rise. The decision tree, which puts numbers on clinical judgement, is in accord with the Oxford group's recommendations on the use of CT scanning made in 1985.

Alternatively, life expectation after CT scanning could be used as the measure of outcome. In this case, the detection of treatable nonvascular pathology (i.e. subdural haematoma, meningioma) would be awarded the full life expectation (assuming negligible surgical mortality) at the average age of onset of the stroke. Life expectations can be obtained from life tables; the expectation for a 70-year-old will be around 15 years. The life expectation for a patient suffering a stroke will be about five years. If these life expectations are used instead of the arbitrary measures of utility, and it is assumed that a third of nonvascular pathology is treatable, doing a CT scan for a patient will 'buy' 3.48 years of life, and not doing a CT scan will produce 3.40 years.

The value of a year of handicapped life compared with a year of normal life could be weighted to give a more refined comparison of the decision whether or not to do a CT scan. The principles would be the same.

Aspirin for every stroke patient?

Since 1988, the beneficial effects of aspirin in secondary stroke prevention must be taken into account, and it has been suggested that every patient considered for anti-platelet treatment after stroke should have a CT scan to exclude a cerebral haemorrhage (Consensus Conference 1988). It is argued that without CT scanning it would not be safe to give aspirin because patients with haemorrhagic lesions might get worse.

Decision trees can be used to quantify the utility (or increased value) of the new information that thrombo-embolic strokes are potentially treatable. A second decision tree is shown in Fig. 4.2. The utilities used are again arbitrary, but it is unlikely that there would be great disagreement on their rank ordering. The decision to do a CT scan is rewarded with a far higher overall utility (0.71) than not doing a CT scan (0.245), largely because the 80 per cent of diagnoses of thrombo-embolic stroke are of greater value now that a treatment is available. It can be seen that the decision tree is not

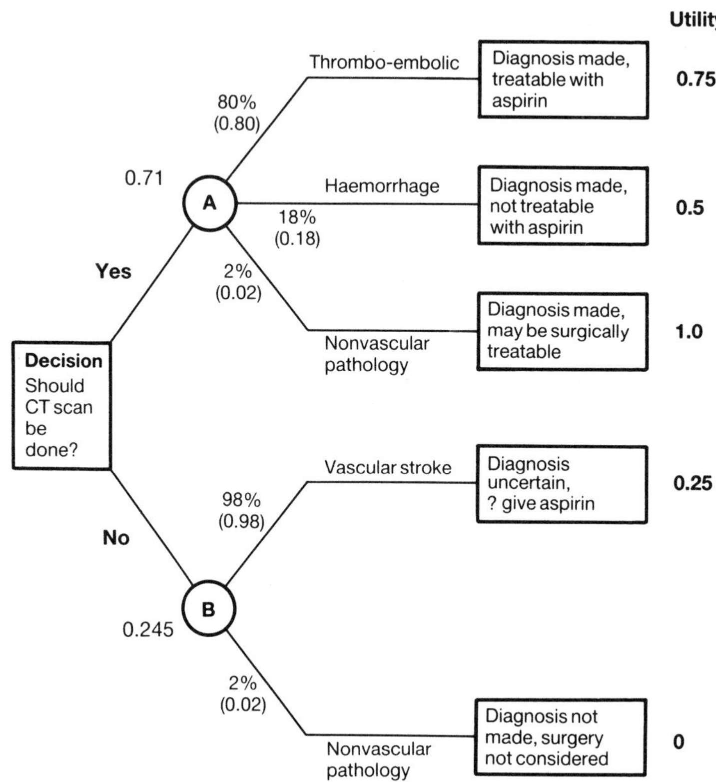

Fig. 4.2 Decision tree: CT scanning and use of aspirin.

very sensitive to the utilities chosen; if the utility of an uncertain diagnosis is given a value of 0.5, the overall utility of the decision not to do a CT scan will rise to 0.49, but this is still a lot less than the value of doing a CT scan.

However, this approach does not consider the wider implications of such a decision. It assumes that CT scanners are available, that resources are infinite and decisions are taken in isolation. It is worth examining the consequences of this strategy of CT scanning and comparing it with other alternatives, in this case, giving aspirin to every one month survivor of stroke, perhaps aided by using clinical scoring and lumbar puncture as diagnostic aids. The consequences can be measured in terms of strokes prevented, lives saved and the costs of investigation and care.

It is necessary to make some assumptions about the incidence of stroke, the costs of CT scanning, the survival of patients with cerebral haemorrhage and thrombosis, the proportion of patients with contraindications to aspirin, the risk of death or disability in patients suffering a haemorrhagic lesion treated with aspirin, and the costs of care among patients misdiagnosed as vascular stroke. Where possible estimates have been derived from the Oxfordshire Community Stroke Project, and all are explicit so the effects of changing the assumptions can be assessed.

Policy 1, which is a policy of CT scanning every patient with a stroke in the United Kingdom, is shown in Fig. 4.3. The UK costs and benefits of this policy can be estimated, as shown in Table 4.1. The costs are approximate and for 1988, and do not include capital costs of CT scanning installation in hospitals without them. The costs measured, together with massive costs for capital development of CT scanning to cover the majority of the country where facilities do not exist, far outweighs the relatively modest benefits.

The cost–benefit ratio of the policy of CT scanning every person with a stroke does not look very advantageous. The cost for every adverse event prevented and nonvascular pathology detected and successfully treated works out as about £20 000 per adverse event (i.e. 967 patients 'benefiting' for around £25 million, which excludes the capital development costs of providing a CT scanner in every district hospital). Cost–benefit analyses merely try to assess the order of magnitude of the relationship and are not meant to be interpreted as absolute indicators of exact costs and benefits. In general, a ratio of cost–benefit of 1:2 is taken to indicate policies that probably should be implemented. The cost–benefit ratio is 4.4 to 1 which makes the policy untenable. Although the reduction in the costs of human life and suffering have not been included in the benefits of the policy, a cost per patient of around £20 000 (i.e. £25.2 million less £6.75 million divided by 967 patients) would have to be assumed for the cost–benefit ratio to equal 1:1. The many assumptions about reductions in costs of care made in these calculations are not particularly sensitive to changes in the estimates because of the overwhelmingly high cost of CT scanning.

A further use of this sort of analysis is to compare the effects of one policy with another and examine the costs per unit of benefit.

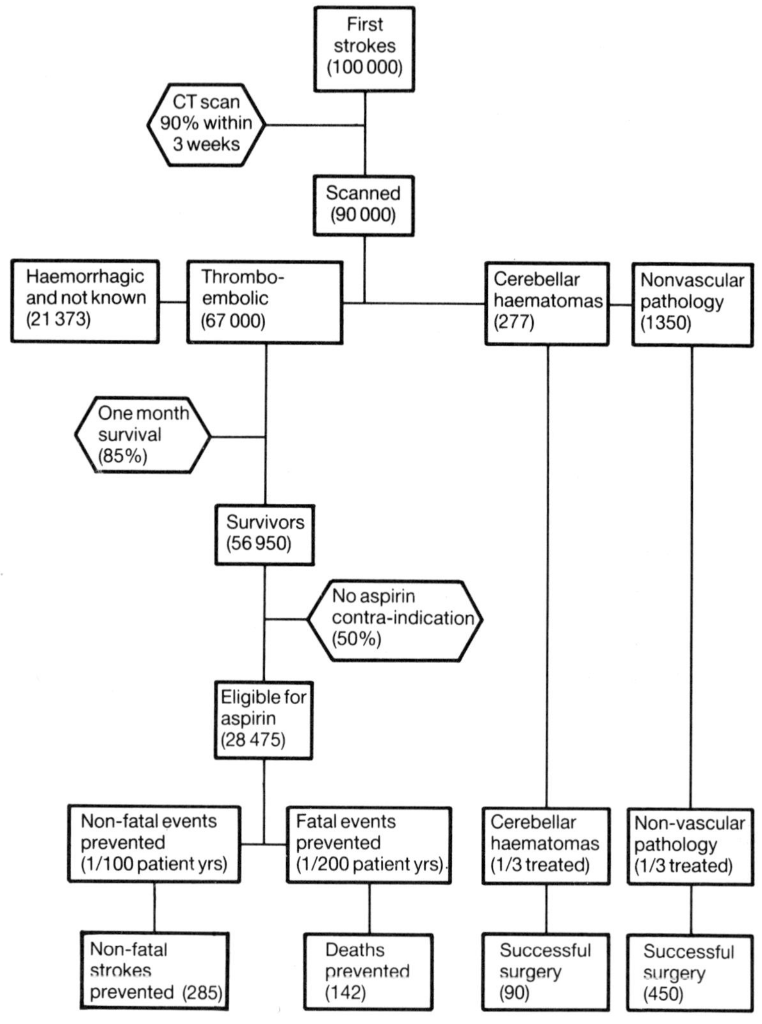

Fig. 4.3 Policy 1: all strokes CT scanned and treated with aspirin if thromb-embolic.

Table 4.1 Costs and benefits of Policy 1: CT scanning of all patients and treatment of those with thrombo-embolic stroke with aspirin

Costs	
Costs of CT scanning (£250 per scan, excludes capital investment)	£22 500 000
Costs of surgery and rehabilitation for those with nonvascular pathology (450 + 90) (£5000 per patient)	£2 700 000
Benefits	
Costs of non-fatal strokes prevented:	
Acute care (285):	
Hospital care (£100 per day for 28 days, for 75% admitted)	£599 200
Community care (£10 per day for 28 days for 25% kept at home)	£19 880
Long-term costs:	
Institutional care (£30 per day for 1 year for 10%, 29 patients)	£317 550
Community care (£10 per day for 1 year for 20% (57) with chronic disability)	£208 050
Costs of suffering to patient and family:	?
Costs of fatal strokes prevented (142):	
Hospital costs (£100 per day for 14 days with 75% admitted)	£149 800
Community costs (£10 per day for 14 days with 25% at home)	£4900
Loss of life	?
Costs of misdiagnosis prevented (450 + 90):	
Subdural haematomas, etc. (£30 per day institutional care for 1 year for 75%)	£4 434 750
Loss of life	?
Total costs (excluding loss of life, effects on family, etc.):	**£25 200 000**
Total benefits (excluding loss of life, effects on family, etc.):	£5 734 130

Cost–benefit ratio: £25.2 million to £5.7 million, i.e. 4.4:1.

In this case, an alternative policy (Policy 2) might be to give aspirin to every stroke patient surviving the first month without using CT scanning in an attempt to exclude cerebral haemorrhage. The consequences of this approach are shown in Fig. 4.4. Obviously treatable nonvascular pathology will not be detected and will lead to costs, and some patients may die or be disabled because they are wrongly treated with aspirin and will suffer an exacerbation of their cerebral haemorrhage. It is difficult to estimate this risk precisely but the UK-TIA Study Group (1988) showed a two-fold increase in risk of fatal haemorrhage among aspirin-treated patients (around two deaths per 1000 patient years of aspirin treatment versus 0.9 deaths per 1000 patient years of placebo treatment).

On a straightforward comparison of deaths and strokes prevented versus nonvascular pathology missed and haemorrhages caused by aspirin, the policy is not advantageous with a ratio of 1:1.2 (i.e. 446 events prevented versus 546 adverse events). The costs of the policy will be much cheaper because the large CT scanning costs are avoided as shown in Table 4.2. Although the policy looks bad because so many patients were misdiagnosed, it is quite likely that a proportion of these patients with tumours and subdural haematomas will be diagnosed eventually without a policy of CT scanning every stroke. Moreover, the two types of event are not strictly comparable: many of the patients suffering a misdiagnosis will die fairly rapidly from untreatable brain tumours whereas the strokes prevented may lead to much longer survival and associated disability. It might be argued that it is fallacious to compare costs and benefits when the cost of human suffering has been ignored. If it is agreed that the cost of suffering is comparable for a patient suffering a stroke and for a patient suffering misdiagnosis, then the cost–benefit ratio of the policy to treat all survivors will be increased by a ratio of 1:1.2 whatever the cost given to human suffering. The cost–benefit ratio for this policy is not in favour of implementation —1.1:1, and the addition of human suffering costs would tend to push the balance in favour of not adopting the policy.

The major reason that the policy is unfavourable is that although aspirin has been shown to reduce the chance of a further stroke, it is not an acceptable drug to use in up to 50 per cent of patients (Sandercock and Warlow 1985). The reasons for non-acceptance of aspirin were not reported but presumably include allergy, past or present history of upper gastrointestinal bleeding, and dyspepsia. If

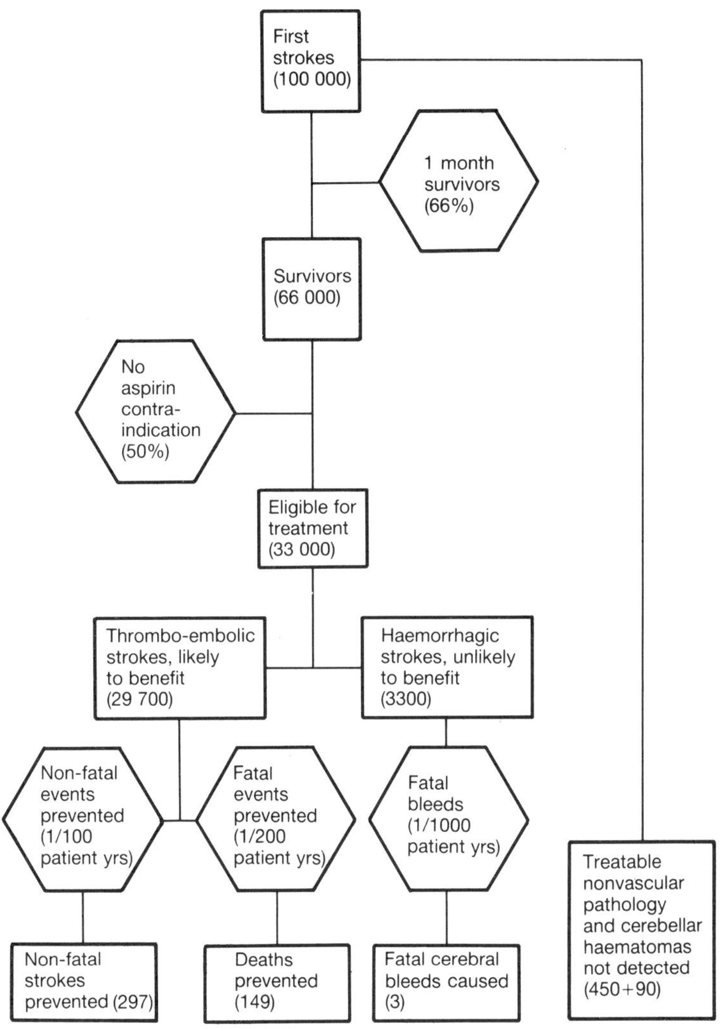

Fig. 4.4 Policy 2: All one month survivors treated with aspirin, without use of CT scanning.

Table 4.2 Costs and benefits of Policy 2: no CT scanning but treatment of all 1 month survivors with aspirin

Costs	
Costs of misdiagnosis: (450 + 90 patients) subdural haematomas, etc. (£30 per day institutional care for 1 year for 75%)	£4 434 750
Costs of three fatal haemorrhages caused by aspirin (£100 per day for 14 days for 100%)	£4200
Costs of suffering and loss of life	?
Benefits	
Costs of surgery and rehabilitation for those with nonvascular pathology avoided (450 + 90) (£5000 per patient)	£2 700 000
Costs of non-fatal strokes prevented (297):	
Acute care:	
Hospital care (£100 per day for 28 days, for 75% admitted)	£624 400
Community care (£10 per day for 28 days, for 25% kept at home)	£20 720
Long-term costs:	
Institutional care (£30 per day for 1 year for 10%—30 patients)	£328 500
Community care (£10 per day for 1 year for 20% with chronic disability—60 patients)	£219 000
Costs of suffering to patient and family:	?
Costs of fatal strokes prevented (149):	
Hospital costs (£100 per day for 14 days with 75% admitted)	£156 800
Community costs (£10 per day for 14 days with 25% at home)	£5180
Loss of life	?
Total costs (excluding loss of life, effects on family, etc.):	**£4 438 950**
Total benefits (excluding loss of life, effects on family, etc.):	**£4 054 600**

Cost–benefit ratio: £4.41 million:£4.1 million, i.e. 1.1:1.

aspirin could be given to a higher proportion of survivors (say up to 90 per cent, which might be feasible with low dose aspirin regimes), the policy to treat all survivors would be marginally advantageous. A further consideration is that because the policy avoids the capital and running costs of providing CT scanners in every district hospital this money could be made available for spending on other services —which is termed an opportunity cost, always assuming the money was there in the first place and the opportunity therefore exists to spend it on something else.

It is not intended that these cost–benefit analyses should be taken too literally. They are presented to demonstrate how an economic approach can be developed from clinical and epidemiological information. Although the analysis is full of assumptions it does force a consideration of the information needed to decide on important health care issues such as the use of CT scanning for stroke patients. Laying out the rows of such tables also helps clarify the consequences of a particular line of action.

In this case, there is a conflict; the clinical decision tree favours the use of a CT scan for every patient because it leads to a higher utility. However, the cost–benefit analysis does not favour CT scanning because of its high costs, but the CT scanning policy leads to twice as many adverse events prevented as the not-scanning policy. This is a familiar problem in clinical medicine, what is good for the individual patient may be very bad for the community as a whole because it does not lead to overall net benefit.

It is possible to combine the costs and utility measures of outcome into a *cost per utility* which may help to clarify whether the use of CT scanning for every patient is a good option. This is shown in Table 4.3.

In this example, the much higher cost of the CT scanning policy

Table 4.3 Comparison of the outcomes of policies of CT scanning all stroke patients vs. not scanning all patients prior to the use of aspirin

Policy	*Utility*	*Cost/Case*	*Cost/Utility*
CT scan	0.71	£252	£355
No CT scan	0.245	£44	£180

is not offset by the higher utility. Life expectation could be used instead of utility measures with a similar result. The addition of the utility outcome has made the CT policy look better; it is now only twice as costly (in the sense of its cost per utility), whereas on a straightforward cost appraisal, it appears to be nearly six times as expensive.

The next step is to decide whether the marginal utility effectiveness obtained by CT scanning is worth the cost investment. This is calculated as the difference in costs of the two policies divided by the difference in utilities (or life expectation) achieved. In this case, the calculation is:

$$(£252 - £44)/(0.71 - 0.245) = £447$$

The marginal cost for one utility unit obtained (or for a year of life if that had been used as the outcome measure) is £447. Whether this is a good way to use resources will depend on comparisons with other policies which may yield a utility (or year of life) at lower marginal cost.

Investigation of the carotid arteries

There is serious doubt concerning the benefits of carotid endarterectomy, both in asymptomatic people and in patients who have had minor strokes or transient ischaemic attacks. Furthermore, there is mounting evidence that the operation is widely, and probably inappropriately performed in the United States. However, proponents of the operation maintain that provided peri-operative risks of stroke and myocardial infarction are low (below 3–4 per cent), then the operation is associated with a reduction in subsequent risk of stroke (Del Campo 1988). The majority of patients operated on in the United States are now over 65 years old, and operations on patients in their high seventies are commonplace. Consequently, it is likely that some elderly patients will be investigated for their suitability for carotid endarterectomy.

The first prerequisite is that the patient is likely to have a lesion that might have been caused by embolus from the carotid arteries. An American audit of the use of carotid endarterectomy among patients over 65 years found that this was often not the case (Loftus *et al.* 1988). The other major problems were that surgeons operated on patients at high operative risk, those with minimal carotid lesions, and those with a carotid lesion contra-lateral to the hemisphere affected.

Non-invasive assessments

The between-observer agreement on the presence of a significant cervical bruit is low, and might easily occur by chance (Chikos *et al.* 1983). The accuracy of a cervical bruit in detecting significant stenosis is also very low, with both false-positives and -negatives. Clinical examination is unreliable, consequently in fit patients presenting with transient ischaemic attacks (TIAs) or with minor strokes of presumed embolic pathogenesis, and if safe carotid endarterectomy can be assured, it is necessary to consider investigation.

Use of doppler ultrasound methods can be considered, and has a likelihood ratio of around 9 for the presence of lesion, and of 0.11 for the absence of a lesion when compared with carotid angiography (Sox *et al.* 1988). The chances of a treatable carotid lesion in patients with carotid TIAs or minor strokes is around 40 per cent (Warlow 1987). A positive ultrasound study will therefore lead to an increase in the probability of the patient having a treatable lesion to 86 per cent, or a reduced probability of 7 per cent if the ultrasound is normal. This and other non-invasive methods of assessment may be less accurate than suggested by the likelihood ratio because only those patients with apparent lesions tend to be investigated with angiography and the investigations depend very much on skill.

Ultrasound investigation will help to avoid carotid angiography in patients with negative results if it is accepted that around one-tenth of these patients may have treatable lesions that will be missed. Those with a positive result will then require carotid angiography to decide whether a potentially operable lesion is really present. Given the uncertainty about the risks and benefits of carotid endarterectomy, and the risks of carotid angiography it is wise to screen potential patients for carotid angiography with ultrasound provided good quality studies are possible. Doing this reduces the number of patients placed at risk from angiography.

Carotid angiography

This technique is probably becoming more accurate with digital subtraction, but reported estimates (compared with operative findings) of sensitivity and specificity in detection of ulceration are only 73 per cent and 63 per cent, a likelihood ratio of 1.97 (Chikos *et al.* 1983). Detection of stenosis is probably more accurate although patients considered to have no ulceration or less than 50 per cent stenosis on angiography are very unlikely to be operated on and consequently the correlation with operative findings in these patients cannot be made. Certainly a positive carotid angiogram (i.e. 50 per cent or greater stenosis and/or ulceration) will increase the probability that an operable lesion is truly present to at least 90 per cent, provided that an ultrasound examination is done initially. This will reduce the chances of operating on patients with apparent rather than real lesions.

Carotid angiograms are subject to disagreement in their interpretation even when broad groups (such as <10, 10–49, 50–99, 100 per cent stenosis) are used. Under these circumstances and with uncertainty about the benefits of surgery, together with evidence of widespread misuse of carotid endarterectomy, it is essential that angiograms are reviewed by a panel of both surgeons and physicians prior to making a decision about operation.

Lumbar puncture

This procedure has two main uses: first to diagnose infection (meningitis, syphilis) in patients who may present with signs suggestive of a stroke. Secondly, to distinguish sub-arachnoid haemorrhage and primary intra-cerebral haemorrhage from a cerebral infarction. With the advent of CT scanning, and because of the danger of tentorial herniation following lumbar puncture in patients with unsuspected mass lesions, this latter indication has fallen into disuse.

The use of subcutaneous heparin after stroke in an attempt to prevent deep vein thrombosis and pulmonary embolus is of particular concern. The small trials that suggest such treatment is useful in the first week of a stroke did not require exclusion of cerebral haemorrhage by CT scanning. Although no complications due to bleeding or worsening of neurological impairment occurred, the studies were too small to give adequate estimates of the risk of giving subcutaneous heparin to patients without first excluding those with haemorrhagic strokes. The use of lumbar puncture to exclude haemorrhage for this purpose should be avoided because if anti-coagulation (even with subcutaneous heparin) is given after lumbar puncture there is a risk of producing a haematoma around the site of the LP which may lead to paraplegia (Ruff and Dougherty 1981).

With increased interest in the use of anti-platelet agents after minor thrombotic strokes, the use of lumbar puncture to exclude cerebral haemorrhage might be thought helpful in centres without access to CT scanning, since it has a high specificity and variable sensitivity, ranging from 72 to 90 per cent (Harrison 1980; Britton *et al.* 1983). It is possible to construct a decision tree for the use of lumbar puncture in deciding whom to treat with aspirin, as shown in Fig. 4.5. At circle A1, the probability of a positive result (i.e. haemorrhagic or xanthochromic tap) is 14 per cent, and of a negative result, 86 per cent. The circle A2 shows the true positive probability (i.e. the sensitivity, which is 72 per cent), and the false-positive probability (i.e. 1-sensitivity). At circle A3, the true negative probability (i.e. the specificity, which is 95 per cent) and false-negative probability are used. Once again arbitrary utilities are used to calculate the overall utility of either decision. The balance is clearly in favour of doing a lumbar puncture. The tree could be made more complicated by including the small risk of coning, which is probably less than 1 in 1000 and may actually be balanced by the small benefit of diagnosing unsuspected meningitis or neurosyphilis.

The decision tree favours doing a lumbar puncture largely because of the high probability that a clear CSF will be found which will lead to the possibility of treatment with aspirin, but a very small chance of treating a haemorrhagic stroke with aspirin inadvertently. The practical problems with such a policy would need to be examined before it could be recommended.

Summary

1. The currently recommended criteria for performing a CT scan are for patients with an atypical clinical course, young patients, where there is diagnostic doubt, and when anti-platelet or anticoagulant therapy is to be started. None of these criteria is supported by evidence that they lead to benefits that outweigh costs.

2. Clinical decision trees may be a useful adjunct to weighing the risks and benefits of particular courses of action. For example,

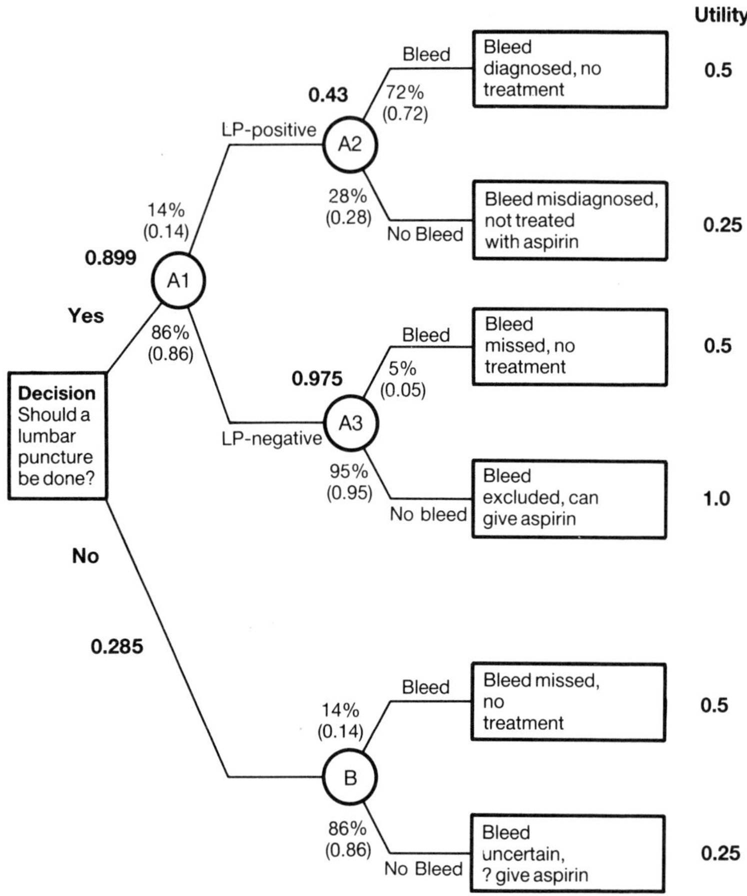

Fig. 4.5 Decision tree: use of lumbar puncture (LP) to decide who to treat with aspirin.

lumbar puncture rather than CT scanning to distinguish haemorrhagic from thrombo-embolic stroke may be a more cost-effective method of deciding whom to treat with aspirin.

3. Combining measures of outcome may be a useful way of deciding between different policies, particularly when there is conflict between the effects of the policy on each outcome.

5 Severity

Is it a bad stroke? The severity of disease can be described in many different ways, ranging from the patient's perception, the degree of physiological disturbance, the consequent disability, and handicap caused, to the burden on society (Stein *et al.* 1987). The severity of a stroke may be assessed in terms of the amount of brain damaged, the size of the lesion(s) demonstrated on CT scanning, or the number and severity of the neurological impairments. At the level of disability, the severity of a stroke may be measured by ability to walk, the ability to climb stairs, or the ability for self-care. At the level of handicap, severity may be measured by impact on work, enjoyment of usual sex life, or social engagement. The aetiological and pathogenetic differences between types of stroke, together with the wide range of possible consequences, make a simple classification of severity difficult.

Impairment, disability, and handicap

A useful model that has gained wide support is the World Health Organization's classification of impairments, disabilities, and handicaps (WHO 1980). It is tempting to consider that a linear relationship exists between each of these markers of severity (e.g. motor impairment leads to difficulty walking outdoors, which in turn leads to the handicap of not being able to go to meet friends). In practice it is much more likely that many factors, such as personality, intelligence, and wealth will operate to either reduce or increase the impact of disease. The distinction between disability and handicap may seem unnecessary, but the former is concerned with ability to carry out tasks, and the latter with the much wider concept of living a role, such as parent, worker, or member of a family.

Impairments due to stroke may lead to disability and handicap, but it is possible for impairments to lead to handicap without disability intervening. For example, a stroke may resolve leaving no disability but leads to the loss of livelihood—a severe handicap—

because the patient's driving licence is taken away. Similarly, some impairments may cause disability but no apparent handicap. In such a case, a stroke may lead to poor balance causing difficulty in climbing stairs—a disability, but the provision of a stair lift permits the patient to continue leading the same sort of life as before the stroke occurred. Not all impairments lead to disability or handicap. An upper quadrantic visual field loss would lead to no disability or handicap for most patients, but for a keen squash player is a disastrous disability and handicap. Finally, patients may suffer with disabilities and handicaps that are due to other pathological processes, unrelated to the stroke, which compound the effects of a stroke.

The WHO impairment, disability, and handicap model is not a complete description of the effects of a disease as it ignores the burden of disease on the family and society. The concept of impairment needs to be widened to accommodate the concept of biological (i.e. anatomical, physiological, and psychological) severity. The biological severity and degree of impairment caused by a stroke are not very useful indicators of severity because no one single marker (e.g. analogous to grading and staging for specific cancers) exists that covers the spectrum of impairments that can result from a stroke. Furthermore, multiple problems which are common amongst older stroke patients cannot be accommodated.

Measures of disability, particularly activities of daily living scales, have gained in popularity as indicators of severity because of a notion that they form a common pathway through which the effects of several, diverse impairments, together with coexisting diseases, express their combined effects. Disability measures are distinct from the level of cell or organ, and are relevant to the aims of rehabilitation and of patients themselves.

Disability measures are thought suitable for a wide variety of purposes, including improving confidence in assessing disability, improving communication between professionals, improving identification of problems, and as a means of standardization of clinical methods (Wade and Collin 1988). In addition, disability measures of severity may be helpful when making comparisons between different diagnostic groups, for epidemiological and health care delivery studies, and to monitor progress clinically. However, even measures that are widely used, such as the Barthel scale (Mahoney and Barthel 1965) and the Katz scale (Katz *et al.* 1963), suffer with problems that need to be overcome. Most scales suffer from 'ceiling' and 'floor' effects that lead to patients with more extreme severities of stroke to either score at the top or bottom of the scale, thus reducing sensitivity to change. Allied to this problem, most scales are not complete descriptors of activities of daily living and are made up of very low-order activities.

Measures of handicap are potentially of greater value to patients who hope to minimize the effects of illness on their lives. Unfortunately, comparatively little effort has gone into this area, in part because of the diverse meanings of the term handicap, and the need to view handicap in terms of individuals and their immediate environment. In practice, much rehabilitation is properly concerned with reducing handicap, but because the tools of measurement are not well developed, it is remarkably difficult to demonstrate that much rehabilitation effort is worthwhile. The Oxford Stroke Handicap scale illustrates an attempt to produce a 'global' 5-point handicap rating (Bamford *et al.* 1989). It ranges from 'no symptoms' to 'severe handicap, totally dependent patient requiring constant attention night and day' and was derived from the Rankin scale (Rankin 1957). Although it is suitable for epidemiological purposes, it lacks sensitivity to change and would be less useful for monitoring progress or measuring outcome. Severity of handicap also suffers from the disadvantage of appearing rather a 'soft' measurement, and, therefore, even if improvements occur they may be due to subjective biases rather than real benefits.

The concept of burden of illness is of value in measuring the effects of different types of illness, can accommodate multiple problems in the same patient, can cope with the diversity of stroke, and can be measured in a variety of more objective ways. Indicators range from the financial cost of an episode of illness, the number of days in hospital, the days of work lost, but can also include the emotional and social effects on the family. However, burden of illness indicators do not correlate directly with other measures of severity, particularly biological/impairment measures. For example, a stroke causing minimal motor paresis with early recovery may lead to a major burden of illness in some patients who embrace the sick role so completely that their families and work suffer. At the other extreme, a stroke damaging most of the brainstem of an elderly patient with no relatives may lead to a very rapid death which will cause a very small burden of illness to society.

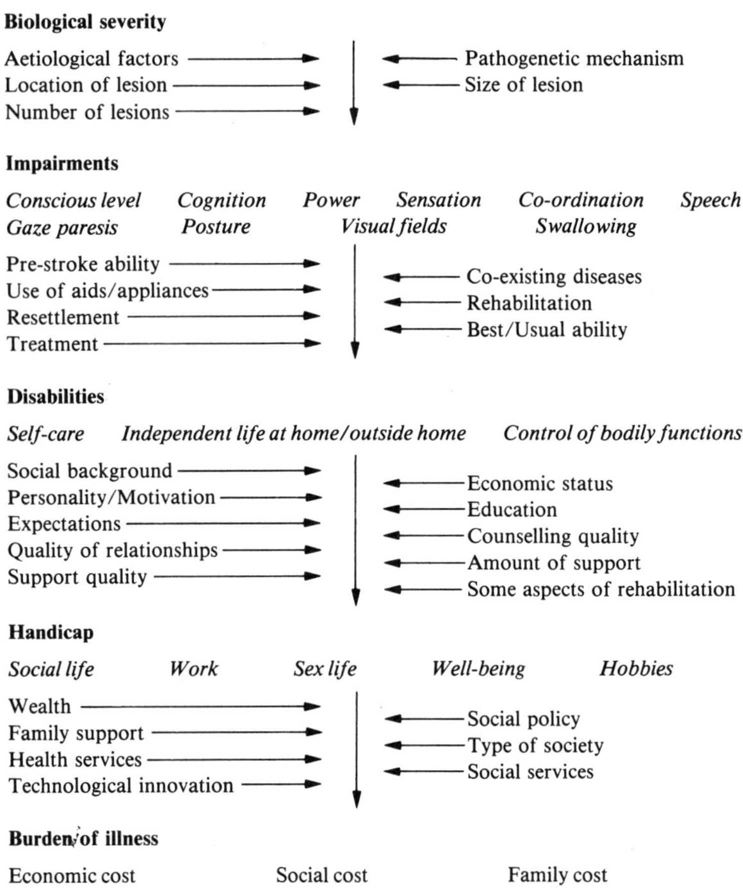

Fig. 5.1 The relationships between impairment, disability, and handicap.

Each of these levels of severity (biological/impairment, disability, handicap, burden of illness) is affected by other factors which explain in part why the relationship between each step in the hierarchy is not direct. Figure 5.1 shows some of these factors.

Severity measures appear complicated enough, but whatever level or type of severity is considered indicators are not likely to be dichotomous (i.e. severe, not severe) nor are they one-dimensional. For example, the duration, treatability, prognosis, and intrinsic 'nastiness' of indicators of severity may all need to be considered depending on the reasons for measurement. Moreover, severity is not a static attribute of an illness but changes with time, and methods of aggregating severity measures over time are needed. Ageing also has an impact on severity measures, as the same biological or disability level of severity will have different consequences and implications at different ages. Finally, it is important to be clear whose value systems are used to decide on which measurements of severity of stroke are relevant. It should not be assumed that professional views of what is severe or important illness are the same as the views of patients, relatives or friends.

Reasons for measuring severity

Prediction

The heart of the question: 'Is it a bad stroke?' is to do with prognosis of individual patients. The question can be rephrased as: 'Which biological features, impairments, disabilities, and handicaps lead to good and bad outcomes?' The relationship between indicators of severity and outcome is confused because often the outcome of interest (e.g. ability to walk or use an affected arm, return home, time spent in hospital, survival) may be used also as a measure of severity. A useful approach to this question is to consider severity at different points in the natural history of the stroke. At onset, prediction of early survival (say, to one month) is of importance together with the likely length of time spent in hospital. The best indicators of survival at onset are the level of consciousness over the first 24 hours, urinary incontinence persisting for a week, gaze paresis, and impairment of swallowing (see Chapter 9 on mortality). Early predictors of discharge from hospital within one month include the degree of arm and leg weakness, conscious level, continence of urine, and age (Barer and Mitchell 1989).

Later, different clinical features of severity are likely to be more important because of the deaths of the most severely affected patients. In a series of patients included in a trial (and therefore not truly representative of all stroke patients admitted to hospital), mobility, age, dressing ability, continence of urine, and power in the affected limbs assessed at one month all contributed to prediction of discharge at three months (Barer and Mitchell 1989). In a more representative series, it is probable that pre-stroke ability and cognitive impairments would also have an impact on early discharge.

The point that deserves emphasis, is that no matter how many severity indicators are measured prediction is not sufficiently accurate to determine management of an individual patient. Measurements made at onset of the stroke will correctly predict one month survival or discharge from hospital in two-thirds to three-quarters of cases. The rest will be wrongly assumed to have a poor prognosis. As time passes, the accuracy of prediction will improve, so that by one month measures of severity will correctly predict discharge from hospital by three and six months in four-fifths of cases (Barer and Mitchell 1989). Nonetheless, it is not possible with present severity indicators to give clinical guidance about which patients should receive rehabilitation and which patients should be resettled in institutions. The best that can be done is to continue with rehabilitation efforts in all survivors until it is self-evident that a good outcome will not be achieved. Although this may mean that resources appear to be wasted on patients who stand no chance of achieving an outcome like discharge from hospital, it is possible that the ability of such patients may improve, that complications of stroke may be less likely to occur, and that the morale of patients and relatives might be sustained. All are reasonable outcomes in themselves.

It is necessary to measure the extent to which rehabilitation does or does not improve disability and reduce complications of stroke among patients who eventually require institutional care. Without such evidence it will be difficult to support present customs of continued rehabilitation until the need for institutional care is obvious in the face of ever tighter financial constraints and limited rehabilitation skills.

The target for the future should be the development of severity measures that are reliable, easy to use, and predict important outcomes with much higher accuracy. It is vital that representative series of patients are used for this purpose, and that predictions are assessed in two independent series of patients to improve the validity of severity measurement. It would also be helpful if more clinically relevant groups (such as, alive at three months, but severe weakness of limbs) of patients were analysed in the manner of

Barer and Mitchell, rather than the continued use of pooled analyses of consecutive series of patients.

Comparison

Indicators of severity are of use when making comparisons between groups. Often, it is desirable to be able to decide whether a treatment given at one centre is worth trying somewhere else. The extent to which the new treatment is worthwhile may be determined (to some extent) by the type of patients seen, and in particular by the severity of strokes suffered by patients. A severity measure can therefore be used as a control for any differences in the case mix treated in a particular place. The simplest way to apply this in practice is to make comparisons only between stroke patients suffering similar types of stroke. For example, if two hospitals had different one month discharge rates for stroke patients, the explanation might be that one hospital had developed a superior acute treatment strategy for stroke. An alternative explanation is that the treatments are identical, but that the severity of strokes seen at each place is different. To control for differences in severity, simple indicators are likely to be the only measures routinely available. In this case, comparisons of patients grouped by their conscious level on admission to hospital could be made. Any differences in one month discharge rates are then more likely to be due to differences in acute treatment practices in the two locations.

Targeting

A further use for simple measures of severity is in targeting of treatments. The concept of triage has been used successfully in a trial of a stroke unit to select patients likely to survive the acute stroke and require rehabilitation (Garraway *et al.* 1981). Triage requires a measure that can be applied rapidly and with reasonable accuracy so that decisions about treatment can be made quickly. In such cases level of consciousness is likely to be the best indicator to use. But even this apparently simple measure can be difficult to apply in practice. A patient who is drowsy on admission has impaired consciousness but may survive the acute phase. A patient who is deeply unconscious and unresponsive to painful stimuli is highly unlikely to survive the acute phase, and the decision to give supportive treatment, such as intravenous fluids and antibiotics, must be made with this knowledge. Whether supportive treatments given to unconscious patients result in longer survival in a disabled state is not known. However, because most early deaths are due to primary brain damage it is unlikely that supportive treatments have much impact on the natural history of the disease process.

Despite much information about prognosis and predictors of good and poor recovery (see Chapter 12 on recovery), it is remarkably difficult to decide which patients should be given high levels of rehabilitation (or be placed on a stroke unit) early in the course of a stroke.

Selection of patients who will benefit most from rehabilitation is a desirable reason for targeting scarce resources. Such thinking clearly prejudges whether rehabilitation makes any difference to recovery, but given that these services exist (and some evidence to support their use can be found, see Chapter 7), methods of selection are required because in many hospitals there are insufficient rehabilitation resources. There is an understandable tendency to put patients who stand a good chance of getting better onto stroke units because of the need to ensure a steady throughput of patients. This becomes a self-fulfilling prophesy; patients selected for their chances of spontaneous recovery will tend to do well. Those not selected because of adverse prognostic signs will tend to do badly. Logically, rehabilitation resources should be directed at those patients who without further treatment will probably have a poor and limited recovery. Further research is needed to define who these patients are.

Outcome

Severity may be an appropriate index of outcome for some interventions, particularly acute drug treatments which aim to reduce the consequences of the initial vascular process. In such cases, it is feasible that treatment will result in a reduction of patients categorized as suffering a severe stroke. However, this approach is likely to obscure treatment effects as most severity indicators are too broad and therefore insensitive to change. Combining various variables that are good indicators of prognosis into an overall score and then measuring the difference in the score at entry into a treatment trial and at a specified time after entry has been used successfully to assess the effects of an acute treatment in stroke (Barer *et al.* 1988*a*). This has the effect of allowing the disparate impairments caused by strokes but has the potential disadvantage of weighting improvements in limb power equally with improvements in speech, for example.

Summary

1. The severity of a stroke may be measured in terms of its biological effects, the impairments, disabilities, handicaps, and burden on society that these produce.

2. A severity measure is not a simple dichotomous variable (i.e. severe stroke vs. not severe stroke). Several dimensions are involved (duration, treatability, associated symptoms, intrinsic 'nastiness'), and the relationship between the levels at which severity may be considered are not necessarily linear.

3. Severity measurements may be used to predict outcome, needs for services, triage patients for management, and permit better comparisons of the results of treatment.

Part II

Management

6 Acute management

Admission to hospital

The first decision at the onset of a stroke is whether the patient requires hospital admission. The reasons for admission are diagnostic ('Is it really a stroke?'), to start rehabilitation early, to give treatment to prevent further strokes, and because of needs for a level of nursing care that cannot be given at home. It is estimated that between 40 and 70 per cent of all strokes in the United Kingdom are not admitted to hospital, but are managed at home by primary health care teams (Bamford *et al.* 1986). In practice, it is remarkably difficult to know how many people are not admitted to hospital, because unless a special project is set up to count them, they are not routinely noted. From estimates of incidence of stroke and numbers of patients admitted to hospital it is possible to make a guess at the proportion of patients kept at home. In Nottingham, this estimate was around 30 per cent kept at home (Barer *et al.* 1984).

Data from the Oxfordshire Community Stroke project has been used to examine the question of why are patients admitted to hospital (Bamford *et al.* 1986). The main reasons for admission in Oxford were severity of the stroke (assessed by degree of motor impairment and level of consciousness at 24 hours after onset), and living alone. These findings were confirmed in a similar study from Bristol (Wade and Hewer 1985*b*). Family doctors gave their major reasons for admission as the need for nursing care (87 per cent), uncertainty about the diagnosis (42 per cent), and to start medical treatment for intercurrent illness (30 per cent). The rapid outpatient and domiciliary service provided by the neurology team was only helpful in 5 per cent of cases in keeping them at home.

It is perhaps surprising that neither the neurologists involved in the study, nor the family doctors viewed early access to rehabilitation services as a relevant reason for admission. It is worth noting that this series of cases had already been 'screened' by the study neurologists and comprised only patients who really had suffered a stroke. Diagnostic uncertainty may be a significant reason for admission if all patients with a possible stroke are considered.

There is no doubt that some severe strokes can be looked after at home, although it is doubtful whether those living on their own can be successfully managed at home. Nor is it certain whether the rehabilitation, education of the patient and family, and medical treatment aimed at preventing a recurrence of the stroke will be adequately managed by a family doctor who, in the United Kingdom, will only see around four or five new strokes each year. A specialist diagnostic service as used in the Oxford project would apparently only reduce the demand for hospital admission by around 5 per cent. A well-organized, rapidly responding nursing team might be able to keep a much higher proportion at home, as in 42 per cent of those admitted this was the sole reason for admission. However, the rehabilitation needs of patients are unlikely to be well served unless co-ordinated multidisciplinary teams are available to assess patients at home, initiate, and monitor management.

Management at home

The Bristol Home Care Study was set up to decide whether providing a multidisciplinary team would reduce the use of hospital resources (to a point where the team would be self-funding), would improve the social and emotional adjustment of patients and their families, and with no detriment to the functional recovery of patients (Wade *et al.* 1985*d*). Patients allocated to the trial were defined geographically in order to avoid problems of individual randomization of patients. This caused problems later on because the trial area appeared to have a higher stroke incidence, which was probably the result of increased ascertainment of milder strokes. The extra strokes in the trial area may have used hospital beds leading to a similar number of bed-days used between control and trial areas. Patients and their relatives did not appear to adjust to the impact of a stroke any better in the trial area, nor was there any difference in patterns of disability.

The multidisciplinary team was mostly comprised of part-time staff, but followed the practices of hospital teams, with weekly team meetings, and division of work between nurses, occupational physiotherapists, and a social worker. The type of staff and style of management needed to treat patients in their own homes compared with hospital is probably different. The team provided around 100 person-hours a week to about five new patients per week, although details of case loads were not given it is likely that about 20–30 patients were current cases requiring attention. This is a substantial work load, and if each profession carried out its assessments, its treatment and monitored progress, there is considerable time pressure. A generic worker, skilled in nursing, rehabilitation, and social work, who would provide most of the care and treatment required (but linked to a hospital team for advice and support) might be a better model of management to assess in the community.

Among the reasons discussed for the failure of the scheme to produce the hoped for outcomes was the sense of competition felt between hospital teams and the new service. The home care team lacked a direct responsibility for the acute management of stroke patients, and therefore was unable to actively encourage use of the service. One of the problems of health service evaluation, highlighted by this study, is that the intervention must be working well (i.e. known, respected, and used) before it can be tested fairly. Controlled trials of health services are difficult to do, or as in this case, difficult to interpret, because the recording of strokes was more efficiently done in the trial area, leading to a potentially biased assessment of the effects of the intervention. The authors found an individual randomized study design was not feasible, and under these circumstances a 'before-and-after' assessment of the changes produced by the home care team might have been preferable to the comparison of trial and control areas. Because of the costs of such studies, it would be worth evaluating new services using observational designs, such as case control studies and before and after comparisons, initially. Services that look promising could then be selected for more reliable testing using large randomized controlled trials.

Centralization of a health district's care for stroke patients has been recommended by an expert panel (Consensus Conference 1988). Responsibility for the care of stroke patients who never come into hospital will remain with the family doctor but a rapid response of stroke services to these patients could be achieved by use of the existing domiciliary visiting arrangements for consultant medical staff, and through domiciliary physiotherapy services with suitably trained, more generic workers.

Reduction in the hospital costs attributable to stroke patients might be achieved by use of early discharge schemes (Townsend *et al.* 1988). These schemes have the advantage of being available to all patients admitted to hospital, and have been shown to be cost-effective.

Acute treatment trials

Stroke is not homogeneous in either its pathogenetic mechanism or in the impairments, disabilities, and handicaps it produces. The desired effects of treatment are ambiguous: survival is desirable, but not if it means survival in an obtunted state. Measurement of changes in the underlying pathophysiology of acute stroke is only recently becoming feasible with Positron Emission Tomography scanning. The potential treatments to be used may be useful in thrombo-embolic disease but positively harmful in haemorrhagic stroke. Consequently, early attempts to determine the effects of treatments for acute stroke have been difficult, confounded by these many problems.

Power

The most frequent problem of stroke trials is that they have been too small. This leads to difficulties in interpretation of trial results for two reasons. First, because stroke is such a heterogenous condition, the findings of a small positive trial may be difficult to apply to individual stroke patients. Secondly, the study, if negative, may be too small to exclude an important treatment effect, that is, it has a low power. This second point often causes confusion, and can be clarified by reviewing Table 6.1.

A treatment that appears effective in a trial may be a rogue result, but the chances of thinking that the treatment is effective when in reality it is not effective (i.e. a false-positive result) is given by the p-value associated with the treatment effect. The conventional statistical approach is to define effects that might have occurred by chance only once in 20 similar trials as significant (i.e. $p = 0.05$ or 5%), and therefore likely to be 'true'.

A treatment that does not produce a statistically significant effect may be true (i.e. the treatment really is ineffective). Altern-

Table 6.1 Comparison of the results of a clinical trial with the true effects of a treatment

Treatment effect in trial	*True treatment effect*	
	Not effective	*Effective*
Not effective	Agreement—not effective	False-negative trial result (power)
Effective	False-positive trial result ($p<0.05$)	Agreement—effective

atively, it may be that the trial is hiding a real effect because it is too small and consistent with a true treatment effect. The best clue that a negative study has low power is to examine the 95 per cent confidence intervals of the differences in outcome between treated and control groups, and then to ask whether the upper limit includes an effect that would be clinically useful. If it does, then the trial should not be interpreted as indicating the treatment is ineffective.

As stroke is such a common disease even small treatment effects (of the order of 10 per cent improvements in outcomes) may be useful if considered in the context of a whole health district or country. For example, a treatment that produced a 10 per cent reduction in mortality (e.g. from 30 per cent one month mortality to 27 per cent one month mortality, a difference of 3 per cent, but a reduction of 3/30 = 10 per cent) among the 100000 first strokes in England and Wales, would lead to a saving of 3000 lives.

The catch is that to detect such small differences very large trials are needed. Trials of small numbers of patients, if negative, will only be able to exclude very large treatment effects. In cases where the risks of treatment are very high, a small trial may be adequate because the benefits of treatment will have to outweigh the risks. For example, trials of thrombolytic therapy in acute stroke may be small (tens rather than hundreds or thousands of patients) because the risks of treatment are likely to be high. In such cases, treatment would have to produce a major benefit, and would therefore be detectable in a relatively small trial.

Various charts and tables are available to determine how many subjects are needed to ensure a trial has adequate power to detect important differences. These charts do not decide what is an 'important' difference, and this requires clinical judgement together with an appreciation of the numbers of patients who will have to be treated to obtain a single beneficial outcome (e.g. life saved, recurrent stroke prevented). In general, trials of treatment require several hundreds or even thousands of subjects in each group if the outcome of interest is survival (or a dichotomous improvement vs. not improved).

Which measure of outcome?

Extensive trials are expensive, and one way around this is to measure an intermediate outcome that can be measured more precisely but is related to the outcome of chief interest. For example, a small trial designed to measure the rate at which cerebral oxygen metabolism recovers in patients given a new drug will have sufficient power to detect an important difference because the number of subjects required is determined by the variance of the outcome measured.

This approach has been used to test the effects of beta-blockade on acute stroke (Barer *et al.* 1988*b*). Changes in a neurological score (comprising conscious level, speech impairment, orientation, response to a command, visual fields, gaze paresis, swallowing difficulty, motor impairment, and sensory impairment) were compared from trial entry to one week and one month. A patient whose orientation improved would gain one point, a patient whose conscious level deteriorated would receive a minus point, and a patient who died would also receive a minus point for each neurological impairment measured.

Unless deaths are counted into other neurological and functional outcomes imbalance between treated and control groups can occur. With days spent in hospital, patients who have died may be counted as contributing the maximum number of days of follow-up. With discharge from hospital, those discharged and those who have died should be counted together as having a 'bad' outcome. The tactic of counting death as equivalent to the worst outcome amongst survivors ensures that the balance achieved by randomization is not upset, and therefore that comparisons remain valid.

Survival and time spent in hospital, and other intermediate outcomes (such as neurological impairments, cerebral blood flow) are only part of the recovery process. The use of activities of daily living indicators and quality of life measures has been put forward as complementing the usual outcome measures (Sandercock 1987*b*). However, the more complex the outcome measures, the more difficult it is to ensure that they are reliably applied to the large numbers of patients needed for trials of treatment. Acute drug treatments that do not have an impact on simple outcomes, such as mortality and hospital bed-days, but appear to have an impact on quality of life or activities of daily living will be unusual, and most probably not due to genuine treatment effects but to imbalance in treated and control groups. As a general principle it is wise to use outcomes that are closely related to the type of treatment given. For example, quality of life outcomes are best reserved for interventions aimed at improving quality of life.

Explanatory vs. pragmatic designs

There are two main trial designs, the explanatory and the pragmatic (Schwartz and Lellouch 1967). Explanatory trials aim to answer the question: 'If patients with a particular condition receive treatment *X*, do they do better than those receiving placebo?' With a pragmatic trial the question is: 'Does a treatment policy of giving drug *X* lead to a better outcome than a treatment policy of giving placebo?' The major difference between the two questions is concerned with the handling of the patients who do not receive a full course of the treatment, and those who leave the trial for other reasons. They may be excluded from the analysis if the trial is explanatory, and are included in the analysis if the trial is pragmatic.

Explanatory trials have an appealing logic; patients who do not get the drug (or the full regime) should not be included in the analysis. This logic is flawed because once some subjects are left out of the analysis, the balance between treatment and placebo groups obtained by careful randomization is lost. This means that any differences in outcome between treated and placebo groups may be due to real effects of treatment, but may also be due to bias in prognosis between the groups. For example, intolerance of mild side-effects of a trial drug may be associated with cognitive impairment following a stroke. Leaving out the poor compliers will lead to fewer cognitively impaired subjects in the treatment group.

The placebo group will have a relative excess, and not surprisingly, a worse outcome on most measures. Thus, the drug will be assumed to be effective. Pragmatic trials answer questions that are closer to clinical decision-making, and also allow an explanatory analysis to be conducted (Hampton 1981).

Generalization

Do the patients included in a trial bear any relationship to patients looked after by the majority of clinicians? If trial patients are highly selected, which they often are, then it is highly unlikely that they will be similar to the typical stroke patient. This is a particular problem in acute treatment trials because, ideally, the patients should have neuro-radiology to define the type and location of the stroke, and should not have other pathological processes that might interfere with measured outcomes, and should have treatment started very early in the course of the event so that potentially reversible pathogenetic mechanisms can be influenced, and should be in hospital to ensure uniform assessment, randomization, and other supportive treatment.

The typical stroke patient is old, with numerous other medical and social problems, is often kept at home, never goes near a CT scanner, and if admitted to hospital, is seldom there within the first few hours of the event. Consequently, trials that try to ensure that the patients randomized are as homogeneous as possible may end up by producing a trial result that is of little relevance to the practising clinician—the problem of generalization.

There is no quantitative way to decide the extent to which a trial can or cannot be generalized to the patients seen in different settings. A judgement must be made by the individual clinician. Trialists can help by their descriptions of the patients they actually studied. In particular, the age range of patients studied, the proportion with other medical problems, the setting from which patients were obtained (e.g. community, specialist neurology centre), and details of the patients not suitable for randomization. These non-randomized patients are the key to interpretation of a trial. If their death rate, for example, is markedly different from those included in the trial, it implies substantial selection has occurred, making it less likely that the trial results will apply to the typical case.

Another technique that helps decide the relevance of a trial to other patients is sub-group analysis, particularly if these have been specified in advance rather than produced following inspection of the trial results (data dredging). The sub-groups of importance are generally male/female differences in outcome, age effects, and stroke severity effects.

Randomization

Balancing out the factors that have an influence on outcome after stroke is important if a valid comparison is to be made between treated and placebo groups. If we possessed complete knowledge about the prognosis of stroke, then a case could be made for allocating patients to treatment groups according to such knowledge. Randomization is simply a method for balancing out both known and unknown factors that may have a bearing on the outcome of interest. The effect of chance dictates that two groups allocated at random should only differ to an extent determined by chance variation.

However, it is possible for simple randomization to go wrong when chance leads to large imbalances between groups. An example of this effect was an early trial of the use of steroids to reduce cerebral oedema (Mulley *et al.* 1978). Nearly twice as many subjects unconscious to the point of being insensitive to pain were randomized to the placebo group. This imbalance is surprising and is statistically unlikely to be a chance occurrence. In this case, although the treatment groups were poorly balanced the bias was weighted in favour of the treatment group having a good outcome, but an insignificant result was obtained.

As conscious level is such an important prognostic variable in acute stroke, this is a good reason for using it to stratify allocation to treatment groups. Patients should be split initially into those with a good prognosis and those with a poor prognosis. Randomization plans for each group, or stratum, should then be applied which will ensure that major imbalances do not occur.

Consistency

A single positive trial result will not alter clinical practice, nor should it. It might be a fluke result, it might only apply to a highly selected group of patients, or other deficiencies in the trial design (e.g. short follow-up, losses and withdrawals, small sample size,

Table 6.2 Mechanism of action of various drugs used in the treatment of acute stroke

Mechanism	*Drug*	*Source*
Reducing oedema	Steroids	Anonymous (1987*b*)
	Barbiturates	Sila and Furlan (1988)
	Glycerol	Bayer *et al.* (1987)
		Sandercock (1987*b*)
Improving blood flow	Haemodilution	Scandinavian Stroke Study Group (1987)
		Italian Acute Stroke Study Group (1988)
	Vasodilators	
	Nimodipine	Gelmers *et al.* (1988)
	Naloxone	Baskin and Hosobuchi (1981)
	Prostacyclin	Martin *et al.* (1985)
	Naftidrofuryl	Steiner and Rose (1986)
	Vasoconstrictors	
	Beta-blockers	Barer *et al.* (1988*b*)
	Theophylline	Britton *et al.* (1980*b*)

Table 6.2 (*cont.*) Mechanism of action of various drugs used in the treatment of acute stroke

Mechanism	*Drug*	*Source*
Reducing neuronal metabolism	Beta-blockers	Barer *et al.* (1988*b*)
	Naftidrofuryl	Steiner and Rose (1986)
	Barbiturates	Safar (1980)
	Hypothermia	Thomas (1984)
Thrombus directed therapy	Anti-platelet agents	
	Aspirin	Gant (1987)
	Oxypentifyline	Mills and Smith (1972)
	Anti-coagulants	Weksler and Lewin (1983)
	Streptokinase	Sloan (1987)
	Tissue plasminogen activator	Koudstaal *et al.* (1988)

side-effects of treatment, etc.) all make most clinicians naturally conservative about trying new treatments on their patients.

A trial of haemodilution in acute stroke highlights the need for a cautious approach to a single trial. An initial report of haemodilution by venesection and infusion of dextran 40 applied to 102 patients admitted to a stroke unit showed clear benefits in the proportion returning home, functional, and neurological recovery rate (Strand *et al.* 1984). Surprisingly these investigators, having obtained a positive result, decided to set up a much larger multicentre trial to test the effects of treatment in a more typical setting than the specialist stroke unit (Scandinavian Stroke Study Group 1987). In all 373 patients were randomized, but this time no benefits of treatment were found in the whole group, or in any sub-group (Scandinavian Stroke Study Group 1988).

The last word on haemodilution is the massive Italian study (Italian Acute Stroke Study Group 1988) which randomized 1267 patients, carried out CT scans on nearly all of them, and disappointingly demonstrated no benefits in survival or disability. Sub-group analyses did not pick out any benefits for those treated very early, for infarcts compared with haemorrhages, or for those patients with high haematocrits at the outset.

The message is quite clear—treatments that look like winners must be subject to further evaluation. With increased demand for research funds and a natural human tendency for novelty, it is difficult to ensure that such replicate trials are done.

New treatments

The search for new treatments for acute stroke has been built on an understanding of the pathogenesis of stroke. The main mechanisms that seem important in determining the extent of damage are cerebral oedema, blood flow in the area around the lesion, neuronal metabolism, and thrombolysis. However, efforts to modify these processes have not been successful. Table 6.2 shows some of the drugs that have been tried.

Innovative treatments may have risks as demonstrated by the use of tissue plasminogen activator (TPA) in acute stroke (Koudstaal *et al.* 1988) These investigators aimed to enter 10 subjects into an open study of the effects of TPA. However, the first two patients suffered with massive and fatal cerebral oedema leading to premature stopping of the study. The investigators calculated the probability of two consecutive patients developing fatal cerebral oedema as a result of chance alone as 1 in 196. Although their calculations were criticized (Steiner 1989), it is likely that the risk of this complication being due to chance was small. However, given the potential of this treatment it seems unwarranted to stop the study before the agreed 10 patients had been studied. Randomized trials are underway in the United States (Sloan 1987).

It is certainly disappointing that none of these therapies has been unambiguously successful. The more recent studies that appear worth further investigation are glycerol, nimodopine, and naftidrofuryl (Sandercock 1987*b*). The trials needed should be large, use a pragmatic design, and apply simple measures of outcome.

Summary

1. Patients admitted to hospital tend to have more severe strokes and to live alone. The need to investigate patients to exclude diseases that may mimic stroke is not well recognized amongst primary health care doctors.

2. The proportion of stroke patients admitted to UK hospitals varies from 40 to 70 per cent. The chief perceived reason for admission is for nursing care.

3. Admission to hospital may ensure rehabilitation is started early. A single trial of a domiciliary rehabilitation team did not succeed in reducing the use of hospital beds, and consequently was not considered a viable alternative to hospital admission.

4. No current acute treatment is successful in reducing the mortality or limiting the brain damage caused by stokes. Clinical trials have suffered with problems of low power to detect important treatment effects because of small sample sizes, have been analysed in an explanatory manner, and have often studied highly selected patients who are atypical of many stroke patients.

5. Future studies must be extensive, should include patients broadly representative of all stroke patients, should be pragmatic in design, and should measure simple outcomes appropriate to the intervention. These outcomes are usually death, days in hospital, or a functional endpoint, such as independent living.

7 Does rehabilitation work?

The nature of rehabilitation

Rehabilitation is 'about the tertiary response to insult or disease' (Goodwill and Chamberlain 1988), and thus is concerned with the prevention of complications of disease. The effects and complications of stroke are discussed in Chapter 12, but rehabilitation is about more than just prevention of complications. It is concerned with reablement—the restoration to former rights, and resettlement—the use of new or prosthetic environments. The World Health Organization defines rehabilitation as: 'the combined and coordinated use of medical, social, educational and vocational measures for training or retraining the individual to the highest possible level of functional ability'. Using this definition a case could be made for everyone, sick or well, receiving their share of 'rehabilitation'.

The rehabilitation approach involves a multidisciplinary team, comprising the patient, the family, therapists, nurses, social workers, and doctors. Team members assess the patient's disease in terms of impairments, disabilities, and handicaps, together with the burden on the family and local services. Priorities for treatment and goals are then defined with the patient and family, and specific therapy may then be started. Non-specific therapy begins with the assessments, priority and goal setting, which encourage the patient and family to begin to understand the nature of the disease and its effects. Regular team meetings are held to monitor progress towards goals, redefining them if necessary, and starting or stopping specific therapies.

Specific therapies may include the Bobarth approach (Bobarth 1970) which emphasizes the developmental approach to recovery (e.g. the patient must achieve sitting balance before proceeding to standing), together with a normal bilateral, rather than hemiplegic, pattern of movement and posture. Some therapists prefer the Brunnstrom methods which make use of the pathological tonic reflexes to maintain posture and carry out activities. The former method aims to avoid inhibitory pathological reflexes, whereas the latter tries to enhance them. Both methods have their proponents, but neither has been evaluated in placebo-controlled trials, or compared with each other.

Occupational therapists usually adopt a 'practice makes perfect' approach, giving the patient plenty of opportunity to re-learn skills, such as dressing and washing. Some daily living skills may require the temporary or permanent use of aids or appliances, which the occupational therapist is trained to provide. Social workers will often be concerned with the emotional and social aspects of stroke, giving advice on coping with the burden of care, as well as practical advice about financial matters. Rehabilitation may take place in various settings, the acute hospital ward, a stroke unit, a day hospital, an outpatient clinic, or at home.

Evaluation of rehabilitation

Given the complexity of the rehabilitation process it is not surprising that the development of suitable summary outcomes to evaluate the effects of rehabilitation has been slow. The tailor-made, therapist-dependent packages of treatment are also very difficult to standardize. An hour spent with a physiotherapist who has the ability to develop a good rapport may be worth weeks of therapy with another therapist with poor social skills.

Evaluation of rehabilitation has many problems that may be categorized into the following groups: the patients, the interventions, and the outcomes.

The patients

Spontaneous recovery. Stroke patients will either die or recover to some extent. This basic information about natural history is fundamental, but explains why many therapies appear to be effective when studied without a concurrent control group. The before-and-after comparison is a fallacious way of assessing whether a treatment has made a difference because allowance is not made for spontaneous recovery. As before-and-after comparisons mimic the usual clinical approach to treatment, they can be quite persuasive evidence to the scientifically naïve. Even well-established types of therapy, such as the Bobarth approach, have not been studied using randomized controlled trial comparisons. Spontaneous recovery can be best allowed for by making comparisons between groups randomly allocated to one or other form of therapy (or indeed, no therapy if that is an ethical option).

Heterogeneity. Stroke patients may look fairly similar to an untutored eye, but to a therapist the challenge is the uniqueness of each patient. This uniqueness applies not just to the type and location of the lesion causing the stroke, but also to the patient's previous abilities, coexisting diseases, social circumstances, emotional response to the stroke, and aspirations.

Evaluation of effectiveness can cope with this problem in two ways. One is to reduce the sources of variation between patients by selecting only those with a particular type of lesion, affecting a particular part of the brain, causing a particular impairment, and so on. The second way is to study large numbers of patients so that the diversity of stroke and its consequences are well represented. The former approach may be self-defeating because of the limited availability of ideally matched groups of patients to compare. It may have some application in the special case of single-case study designs (see 'Future developments', p. 125). The use of large numbers is a good approximation to clinical practice, where rehabilitation teams do not select patients with very specific problems, but take what comes through the doors and apply their skills.

Numbers. The number of subjects available to be evaluated may be too few, although in clinical practice there always seem to be too many patients requiring attention! As with any attempt to evaluate therapy it is essential that a prior effort is made to calculate the number of subjects that will need to be compared to establish whether the null hypothesis (i.e. no effect of treatment) can be safely accepted if the study produces a negative result (see Chapter 6 on acute management).

Selection bias. A successful rehabilitation team chooses patients that it knows it can help. To a greater or lesser extent rehabilitation leads to selection biases. Selection of patients who are 'motivated' enough to continue attendance at the rehabilitation department will tend to produce better results than trying to treat every patient. Selection of therapists who are particularly 'good' with stroke patients to work on a unit may achieve better results than those of therapists working in other settings or locations.

The best way to overcome the problem of selection of patients is to set up explicit criteria for inclusion in a study of the effectiveness of rehabilitation, and to measure what happens to all those patients who are allocated to the programme, and not just those who finish it. Selection of individual patients for therapy is therefore removed from the therapist's control, and thus removes this potential source of bias.

The intervention

Therapy and therapists. Rehabilitation practice is built on experience with largely untested treatments, depends on interaction between patient and therapist, and between members of the rehabilitation team, and aims to treat the patient in an individualized way. Randomized controlled trials are generally agreed to be the best way of deciding whether an intervention 'works' (Meade 1977; Garraway and Akhtar 1978), but it is difficult to conceive of how a satisfactory trial can be set up when the intervention can be so variable. Rehabilitation does not fit comfortably into the model of a placebo-controlled drug trial. One solution to this problem has been to treat the intervention as a 'black box', assuming that what goes on between patients, therapist, and team will be more or less the same for each patient. The danger with this assumption is that a trial of therapy can turn out to be a trial of therapists.

A further problem with non-standardized therapies is that they will tend to vary over a period of time, and between places. At present Bobarth-orientated physiotherapy is very popular in the United Kingdom, but this will probably wane. Evaluation studies should clearly specify which type of regimen is used, otherwise it will be impossible to distinguish the effects of types of therapy from the more non-specific effects of contact with rehabilitation teams.

Ethics of rehabilitation. This is now a major part of the health services, and despite relatively little scientific evidence of its effectiveness, is assumed to work by both the lay and professional. Consequently, the opportunity to test whether a rehabilitation treatment is better than spontaneous recovery is rapidly disappearing because many people believe that it is now unethical not to offer all stroke patients access to rehabilitation.

At present it is impossible to say whether investment in extra occupational therapists, for example, will result in a net saving of hospital bed-days (that could fund the initial investment). It is not clear whether specific forms of rehabilitation have any merits over and above practice and encouragement. The time-consuming and elaborate assessment and teamwork rituals of rehabilitation teams may be a poor use of time for the majority of patients. Answering questions about the effectiveness of rehabilitation will develop the scientific basis of rehabilitation, and will lead to much greater competitiveness in maintaining and even increasing present resource levels for rehabilitation.

The present position is analogous to the state of medical practice only three decades ago, when the art of medicine was paramount and scientific evaluation of the benefits and risks of treatment was just beginning. In the late 1950s, it would have been unthinkable to advise a patient who had recently suffered a myocardial infarction to start an exercise programme, but now this is commonplace.

The main ethical dilemma faced by rehabilitation teams is whether they are being wasteful of resources in continuing to carry out untested, unstandardized methods of treatment. If there is doubt about the value of a therapy, then it should be put to a scientific test. The other aspect of this problem is that so little is known about what are the important components of rehabilitation. Consequently, it is all too easy to conduct trials prematurely in the development of a therapy.

Dosage and timing of rehabilitation. On average, a stroke patient receives 30 minutes of physiotherapy and 10 minutes of speech therapy a day (Langton-Hewer 1973). A trial of speech therapy after stroke (Lincoln *et al.* 1984) which demonstrated no advantage from therapy over the expected spontaneous improvement in language recovery was fiercely criticized because the amount of speech therapy received was too little, and yet it was exactly what was used in usual clinical practice. Little is known about the optimum amount of therapy, and it is unlikely that the relationship is linear or cumulative.

Of equal importance may be the timing of rehabilitation. Early access to a rehabilitation team may be more important than the actual amount of therapy given. This appears to be shown in the Edinburgh stroke unit trial (Garraway *et al.* 1981), which showed that although stroke unit patients received fewer hours of therapy contact, they achieved independence sooner than medical ward patients. Stroke unit patients were seen by an occupational therapist within one week, whereas medical ward patients were seen by three weeks on average. By contrast, physiotherapy was received within the first week by both stroke unit and medical ward patients. This may mean that early access to the team is important, but it may be that it is the occupational therapy intervention that is crucial. It is important to know which of these inferences is correct, as the resource implications of developing stroke units are rather larger than recruiting extra occupational therapists.

The outcomes

Relevance to therapy goals. Rehabilitation has very wide-ranging goals, and is certainly concerned with more than gaining a level of independence in activities of daily living. Part of the difficulty is that therapists may define their success (or failure) in many different but interrelated ways. Success may be an improvement in an impairment (e.g. the degree of spasticity in a limb, or the range of movement of a joint). It may be recovery of an ability such as walking or dressing, or using the lavatory. Success may be defined as a return home to a spouse who has at last come to terms with illness in the family after much counselling and support; or it may be a patient who looks and feels happy, or at least accepting, of chronic ill-health.

A further confusion is the concept of autonomy, which need not necessarily be related to dependency at all. Very dependent people can be totally autonomous in the control they exert over what happens to them and those around them. Indeed, it might be argued that the role of rehabilitation is to achieve the maximum level of autonomy for a patient, regardless of the degree of impairment and disability suffered.

A useful method of considering the options for outcome measures is to classify them as relating to impairments, disabilities, and handicaps. Given the multiple interventions used in rehabilitation it will usually be necessary to measure more than one outcome. In a review of 50 articles concerned with stroke rehabilitation it was noted that there is an overemphasis on physical self-care indicators, with virtually no attention given to indicators of well-being, quality of life, satisfaction with care, or return to work (Seale and Davies 1987).

Repeatability, validity, and sensitivity to change. Outcome measures must perform well to be of any use. Measurement of any biological variable will show some random variation, but provided this variation is small compared with the effects of therapy that are to be detected then this does not matter. It is important to know how repeatable a measurement is when used at different times on patients who have not changed clinically (within-observer variation), and when it is used by different people (between-observer variation). If observer variation is large relative to possible treatment effects, the measurement will be of little use as an outcome of treatment.

The validity of an outcome measurement is the extent to which it agrees with a superior way of measuring the same outcome. Measurements of disability and handicap do not lend themselves to comparison with a superior method, as the outcome used is usually only one of several methods of assessment, none of which is clearly better than any of the others. In these circumstances, it is useful to examine the extent to which the outcome concurs with other indicators that have some bearing on success or failure. For example, relating a disability measure with lengths of stay in hospital gives an indication that the disability measure is valid (Ebrahim *et al.* 1985).

The sensitivity of a measurement to changing patient abilities or handicaps is an obvious requirement. Broad patient groupings such as the Rankin classification (Rankin 1957) are useful for assessing the severity of strokes seen in a unit, for example, but useless for assessing improvement. Patients may have improved substantially, but not move up to a higher category. The extremes of the scale pose a further trap; patients may improve beyond the limits of the scale, particularly with the widely used Barthel activities of daily living scale (Mahony and Barthel 1965). Equally, the lowest limit of the scale does not correspond with the nadir of disability patients may experience.

Popular outcome measures. Widely used, popular measures have advantages (Wade and Collin 1988). It is claimed that use of a standard measure would improve: the attention given to the subject of disability; communication between staff; problem identification; and would permit different research studies to be compared. These may be more apparent than real advantages. As noted by

Seale and Davies (1987), rehabilitation is concerned with far more than ability in self-care. The Barthel scale, advocated by Wade and colleagues, limits understanding of the scope of disability, the type of problems identified, suffers from marked ceiling effects, and when used routinely in clinical practice can reduce rather than increase communication between rehabilitation team members. The Barthel Scale may not be the 'best buy'.

By far the most important criteria in choosing outcome measures are that they should be relevant to the stated goals of a rehabilitation programme, and should be scientifically tested to ensure repeatability, validity, and sensitivity to change. If the measure chosen is also a widely used, popular measure, so much the better because this will aid others in interpretation of results.

Independent measurement of outcome. If a rehabilitation team has to decide whether its own efforts are worthwhile or not, there will inevitably be a conscious or subconscious desire to see the best side of the service, minimizing any shortcomings. This is a bias that is difficult to avoid without special safeguards. In routine clinical practice it is acceptable for patients and therapists to decide for themselves whether treatment is improving things. When conducting more formal evaluation, this is likely to lead to the expected affirmative answer.

The best way to avoid this bias is for outcome measures to be made by people other than the therapists conducting treatment. This should give more objective results, but cannot be done 'blind' to the patient's treatment status, as the patient knows whether treatment has been given and may tell the assessor. Self-assessments by patients themselves may also be prone to this sort of 'self-deception' bias and consequently are not an alternative to independent assessors.

A further refinement of this method is to ensure that therapists are not informed of the trend that results are taking during the course of an evaluation study. The object of this is to prevent therapists from prejudging the overall outcome and either becoming more or less enthusiastic in their approach.

Studies of effectiveness

The favoured method for deciding whether any treatment, drug or health service, is effective is to conduct a randomized, controlled trial. If the treatment can be made blind to either recipient or provider, and preferably both, the trial removes a powerful source of bias referred to above. Randomized controlled trials are not the only way of studying the effects of treatment, and present major problems for the investigator. The major trials of stroke rehabilitation will be presented in turn, highlighting their strengths and weaknesses. Other methods of evaluation of effectiveness will be covered at the end of this chapter.

Stroke units

Studies of stroke units were among the first trials of the impact of health services on stroke patients. In the United Kingdom, plans to develop stroke units in each health district were put forward in 1974 (Royal College of Physicians 1974). The benefits that stroke units would bring were thought to be:

1. Concentration and co-ordination of scarce resources.
2. Education of staff.
3. Planning of progressive patient care.
4. Initiation of research projects.

The main emphasis in this early report was on the research potential of stroke units and, in particular, the evaluation of whether patients in a stroke unit did better than those having usual care.

By 1982 several stroke units had been established in the United Kingdom (Chest, Heart and Stroke Association 1982). Of 12 units, nine were within departments of geriatric medicine, two were attached to departments of neurology, and one was part of a regional rehabilitation unit. The units ranged in size from 10 to 20 beds, which represented between 0.5 and 1.0 beds per 1000 population aged over 65. All adopted a multidisciplinary team method of working, but most did not use a triage system to select patients. None of the units was responsible for all patients admitted to hospital with stroke. Several units provided relatives support groups, health education, and staff training programmes, as well as research activities.

Stroke units have not been widely adopted, and have provided only a small amount of the direct care of stroke patients. They have had a disproportionate impact on research, probably by providing a base for a nucleus of investigators. Their contribution to improved standards of care for stroke patients is not assessed in any of the trials established to measure their effects.

Four trials of the effects of stroke units have been carried out and all have been comparisons with usual medical ward care. The details of each are summarized in Table 7.1.

When the results of a stroke unit are assessed, although deaths may be inevitable and not affected by rehabilitation, allowance must be made for them (Barer *et al.* 1988*a*). If this is not done the balance produced by randomization at entry may be lost. This can be avoided by combining all bad outcomes (deaths and dependency) and comparing them with good outcomes (independence). This will maintain the initial balance between patients randomized to the stroke unit and to medical unit care. The results of the four published trials are shown expressed in this way in Table 7.2.

The New York study was the earliest and the only one to consider a wider range of outcomes than activities of daily living. Patients were randomized up to two months from onset of the stroke which probably explains the absence of any deaths. Its value would have been enhanced by stating the times at which outcomes were measured.

The odds ratios are a useful way of expressing the size of the effects of treatment. Only the Edinburgh trial found a statistically significant treatment effect—a two-fold increase in good outcomes. The Dover trial suggests a 60 per cent benefit, but with wide confidence intervals that fall below 1.0. The trial is consistent with both a small adverse effect of stroke units and a greater than two-fold improvement in outcome.

The Uppsala trial which found no treatment effect was not a truly randomized design as patients were allocated to each type of care on a fixed rota, which might permit biased allocation of patients. Moreover, there may have been some 'carry over' effects of therapy between the stroke unit and medical wards which were adjacent to each other (Hamrin 1982*a*). This, together with the small trial size, may have reduced the chance of demonstrating a significant benefit from stroke unit care.

Early outcomes (at discharge or three months) for stroke unit care are significantly better than medical unit care when all three studies are pooled. The pooled odds ratio shows that stroke unit

Table 7.1 The effects of stroke units

Place	*No. of subjects*	*Outcomes considered*	*Timing of measurements*
New York, USA (Feldman *et al.* 1962)	42, stroke unit 40, medical unit	Activities of Daily Living (ADL) Motor impairment Intellectual impairment Employment Residence	Initial and final No further details
Edinburgh, UK (Garraway *et al.* 1980*a*,*b*)	155, stroke unit 152, medical unit	ADL Mortality	Discharge or 16 weeks and 1 year
Uppsala, Sweden (Hamrin 1982*b*)	60, stroke unit 52, medical unit	ADL Mortality Mental capacity Motor activity	3 months and 1 year
Dover, UK (Stevens *et al.* (1984)	112, stroke unit 116, medical unit	ADL Mortality Place of discharge Complications of stroke	Discharge, 4 months, 8 months and 1 year

Table 7.2 Early and late outcomes of stroke unit effectiveness studies, expressed as odds ratios, together with 95% confidence intervals

Early outcomes (at discharge or 3 months)

Place	*Stroke unit outcome*		*Medical ward outcome*		*Odds ratio*
	Good	*Bad*	*Good*	*Bad*	
Edinburgh, UK	78	77	49	103	2.1 (1.3 – 3.4)
Uppsala, Sweden	16	44	17	35	0.8 (0.3 – 1.7)
Dover, UK	71	41	60	54	1.6 (0.9 – 2.6)

Pooled odds ratio 1.6 (1.1 – 2.1)

Late outcomes (at 1 year)

Place	*Stroke unit outcome*		*Medical ward outcome*		*Odds ratio*
	Good	*Bad*	*Good*	*Bad*	
New York, USA*	28	15	22	17	1.4 (0.6 – 3.5)
Edinburgh, UK	56	93	52	94	1.1 (0.7 – 1.8)
Uppsala, Sweden	19	41	19	33	0.8 (0.4 – 1.8)
Dover, UK	66	46	54	62	1.6 (1.0 – 2.8)

Pooled odds ratio 1.23 (0.9 – 1.6)

* The outcome used for the New York trial is final residence. No details are given of the timing of measurements, and the published figures do not add up correctly.

care produces a 1.6 times better outcome than medical unit care. This is a substantial and significant treatment effect.

The late outcomes of care show an important but statistically insignificant treatment effect. However, even with a pooled analysis, relatively few patients have been studied and the pooled results show a 23 per cent treatment benefit. Only the Edinburgh trial showed a marked difference between early and late outcomes. This was caused by a deterioration in independence of 19 per cent of patients allocated to stroke unit care, and an improvement of 24 per cent of medical patients. The improvement of medical patients may be explained by the variable timing of discharge outcome measurements. Those medical unit patients who improved later on were discharged very much earlier than the others who did not change between discharge and one year. Consequently, spontaneous recovery after discharge may have accounted for their improvement. All early outcomes should have been measured at a fixed time after the stroke which would have avoided this problem.

The deterioration of the patients in stroke units is more difficult to explain. One possibility is that patients were encouraged to perform at their maximal level on the stroke unit but on discharge fell back to a less active life style. Assessments of independence in functional ability carried out at home, and self-reports of disability, tend to be lower than direct observations carried out in the standard circumstances of a stroke unit (Sheikh *et al.* 1979; Ebrahim *et al.* 1985*b*). The Edinburgh study should have used all the activities of daily living information available rather than a dichotomous independence/dependence catagorization. The scale of the deterioration, together with an account of the specific activities lost by patients, would have allowed a deeper interpretation of the results.

Pooling of the late outcomes indicates a beneficial result of stroke unit care, but with wide confidence intervals. The major problem with stroke unit trials is their small size leading to inadequate power to detect potentially important effects. The trials would have been enhanced if activities of daily living data had been treated as a scale score. Differences in average scores could have been compared which would have given greater precision in estimates of treatment effects.

Acute drug trials aim to influence pathogenetic pathways and consequently only need to consider a narrow range of outcomes—deaths and days in hospital, for example. Rehabilitation trials must measure a wider range of outcomes because rehabilitation is likely to have its effects at the levels of disability, handicap, and on the overall burden of disease (see Chapter 5 on severity). Stroke units may have only a limited impact on motor impairment and disability, the bulk of improvement being due to spontaneous recovery, but might be expected to have a major effect on handicap, quality of life of partner and family, and adjustment to disability. No recent studies have examined such possibilities.

The educational and research benefits of stroke units have not received any formal evaluation. Educational benefit could be assessed by examining the numbers and types of staff trained on the unit, changes in their knowledge, attitudes and skills related to management of stroke patients compared with staff not having stroke unit experience, and whether this influenced their careers. Research benefits could be assessed by recording the number of scientific papers produced by staff working from stroke units. Although several stroke units appear to be very productive (Bristol, Nottingham, Edinburgh, in particular), the Oxford researchers, with a special interest in stroke, have produced a large series of valuable publications from a community register of stroke patients.

Outpatient rehabilitation

Management after the hospital phase of stroke was studied by the UK Northwick Park Hospital team in London. The trial was established to decide whether two different intensities: (1) intensive (4 whole days per week); and (2) conventional (3 half-days per week), of outpatient rehabilitation were more effective than no rehabilitation. The control group received usual care but with the addition of health visitor visits. Although stroke is a common problem finding sufficient patients to include in the trial was difficult, and recruitment of 121 patients took six years. This was largely because of deaths and 'full' recovery which excluded just over half of the 1094 patients initially considered for the trial. Almost a third of the 1094 patients were excluded because they were considered 'too frail' to withstand the highest intensity of outpatient rehabilitation.

It was unfortunate that frail elderly patients were excluded because they are just as likely to benefit from rehabilitation. Numerically they are important, and their inability to cope with an intensive regime was not supported by any evidence. Indeed, experience in geriatric day hospitals shows that 'frail' old people are surprisingly resilient. The authors went on to conclude that the need for rehabilitation of stroke patients is much smaller than formerly realized, and that only 11 per cent (the proportion they randomized) actually require it. In addition to the frail elderly, who require rehabilitation, many of the patients considered to have recovered fully may have had good reasons for continued rehabilitation, because the index of recovery used was competence in self-care activities of daily living. Other higher-order activities such as driving, shopping, using public transport, social activities, and sex life were not considered, and yet may be relevant areas for rehabilitation.

The patients were assessed at entry, three months, and one year, using a modified Barthel activities of daily living scale (Sheikh *et al.* 1979). This had been well tested for repeatability with only small between-observer and within-observer patient variation. Validity was tested by comparison with a cerebral lesion score, which was related to the size of the lesion, but showed only weak correlation. No other aspects of recovery were reported, although measures of motor power were made. Despite the wide-ranging goals of rehabilitation, no attempt was made to examine other outcomes.

The patients randomized were young (average age 63–65 years), two-thirds were men, and most had spent less than a month in hospital. Their average activities of daily living scores were very close to the bottom of the scale (i.e. almost 'independent'), ranging from 21 to 22 with the best score possible being 17. The main findings are shown in the Table 7.3.

The investigators claimed to have shown a 'dose-response' relationship between intensity of therapy and disability outcome. However, the difference between the intensive and conventional

Table 7.3 Northwick Park outpatient rehabilitation study, main results (from Smith *et al.* 1981)

	Intensive *4 d/wk* ($n = 46$)	*Conventional* *3 half-d/wk* ($n = 43$)	*No rehabilitation* ($n = 44$)
Activities of Daily Living score at entry	22.0	21.5	21.1
Improvement in ADL from entry to 3 mths	3.5	2.9	1.5
Improvement in ADL from entry to 1 yr	3.5	2.9	0.6
% deteriorating between entry and 3 mths	2% (−2%–6%)	10% (0.7%–19%)	24% (11%–37%)
% deteriorating between entry and 1 yr	6% (−2%–14%)	11% (0.8%–21%)	23% (9%–37%)

regimes was not statistically significant, nor was the difference between conventional therapy and no rehabilitation. The dose-response relationship might easily be a chance finding. Confidence intervals for the mean values reported would have made this apparent.

The timing of improvement is interesting. Little further improvement occurred in either therapy group after three months. If increased amounts of therapy are really associated with increased functional ability in a dose-response fashion it would be reasonable to assume that the cumulative effects of therapy in the conventional group should have brought them up to at least the three month level of the intensively treated group. This did not occur. The conclusion should be that rehabilitation, regardless of its intensity, appears to have benefits over no rehabilitation over a short time period. The first few months after a stroke are the period of most rapid spontaneous recovery. Early outpatient rehabilitation seems to build on this recovery, but to have no additional effects after this phase is over.

More patients deteriorated in the group not receiving rehabilitation. The differences in deterioration rates at three months and one year were highly statistically significant. Deterioration following stroke is often because of physical or mental ill-health. The investigators do not give the reasons for deterioration, and it seems illogical to attribute deterioration to lack of rehabilitation unless the causes are considered.

Despite the criticisms that can be levelled at this trial it remains the best example of a well-executed trial of rehabilitation in this field. The patients were reasonably homogeneous, the intervention was practical although its components were not specified, assessments were made independently of therapy, and an objective measure of outcome was used. As well as providing positive evidence of benefit, it has paved the way for a much greater understanding of the difficulties in carrying out adequate evaluations of rehabilitation.

Team care

The stroke unit and the outpatient department offer both a geographical location and a team approach to rehabilitation. An alternative way of achieving team care is to provide a visiting team who care for patients on the medical wards to which they are admitted.

A visiting team service is feasible and requires no increase in resources in a district general hospital (Stone 1987). In one scheme, a junior doctor was responsible for registering each stroke patient admitted every day and making appropriate referrals to the rehabilitation team. The team made a weekly visit to each ward to set goals, monitor progress, and discuss treatment. Family counselling has also included in this programme. Rapid referral, individual treatment programmes, and good communication between staff and family were all achieved. Uncertainty remains about whether the investment of time and effort produced commensurate improvements in disability and handicap.

A randomized controlled trial of a similar team approach examined the mortality, activities of daily living, and motor impairment at 5 weeks after the onset of the stroke (Wood-Dauphine *et al.* 1984). Subsequent follow-up has not been reported, but the early results demonstrated a trend towards increased recovery of Activities of Daily Living (ADL) amongst those receiving team compared with traditional care. A surprising finding was that men did better than women, both in survival and recovery. This sex difference was not related to age, marital status, or living alone. Other studies of rehabilitation have not demonstrated such an effect, and it may be that these observations were a chance finding.

Establishing a stroke unit requires a positive commitment of resources which may be difficult to achieve, particularly given the rather limited evaluations of effectiveness that have been conducted. In districts where it proves difficult to set up a unit the team approach is an attractive method of improving some aspects of the organization of care for patients. As experience is gained it is possible that the resources to start up a defined unit will be found, and any problems of staff recruitment and retention, eased. One of the major disadvantages of a stroke unit is the plight of the patient not accepted for rehabilitation (Stevens *et al.* 1984; Stone 1987). It would make good sense for a stroke unit to offer a weekly visiting service to other wards, modelled on the team approach.

Future developments

Refining the therapy

Previous evaluation studies have treated rehabilitation as a uniform therapy and equated the amount of therapy with its duration rather than considering its quality. The components of a rehabilitation programme are complex; some may be vital but other parts may be of less importance. It is necessary to define which components of rehabilitation are responsible for beneficial effects.

Single-case study designs hold great promise for working out which techniques work and which do not. In general single-case studies mimic clinical practice. A patient's abilities are recorded to give baseline data, an intervention is tried and abilities are recorded again, and finally the intervention is withdrawn and further records of abilities made. This is called an A–B–A study design. In any disease with a spontaneous pattern of recovery this simple design will be inadequate since no control for spontaneous recovery is included. This can be overcome by recording a range of baseline abilities, some of which may be influenced by specific therapy and some of which will not. For example, in dysphasia, recovery of naming ability may be improved by a practice regimen, whereas fluency of speech will not. If following a training programme, baseline measures of naming ability improve, but fluency does not, then it is more likely that the beneficial effects are due to therapy. This method is certainly not foolproof. If the natural history of recovery of different aspects of language differs, for example (which it probably does), then a spurious conclusion of effective therapy may be made.

A series of single-case studies showing benefits of similar magnitude in different patients adds further weight to concluding that a therapy is effective. Single-case studies should go a long way to disentangling the effects of rehabilitation. Interventions that require study are Bobarth orientated physiotherapy, bio-feedback training methods, cognitive impairment practice regimes, and counselling.

The single-case design has been used to evaluate perceptual retraining methods commonly used by occupational therapists (Edmans and Lincoln 1989). Therapy was shown to be of no use in a series of single-case studies. Single-case designs are an efficient way of testing potential therapies. Those that look promising should then be subjected to a randomized controlled trial to answer wider questions about the generalizability of the therapy and its cost-effectiveness.

Summary

1. Rehabilitation aims to reduce the handicapping effects of disease by processes of reablement and resettlement. Its scientific study has been limited by the multiple levels at which therapy may have its effects, and the problems of defining suitable outcomes.

2. Evaluation of the effects of rehabilitation has to take into account the spontaneous recovery that occurs after a stroke, the heterogeneity of the impairments caused by strokes, the number of patients needed to make adequate measurements of treatment effects, and the effects of selecting patients for therapy.

3. The nature of therapy itself must be better defined so that the effects of standardized types and amounts of treatment can be compared.

4. Relevant outcomes that are repeatable, valid, and sensitive to change are needed. Rehabilitation has its effects at the handicap end of the spectrum of severity, but suitable handicap outcomes are not well developed.

5. Stroke units appear to have beneficial effects in the early months of recovery, but longer-term benefits are doubtful. The educational and research benefits of stroke units have been ignored in formal evaluations.

6. Outpatient rehabilitation improves performance in activities of daily living among younger patients suffering less severe strokes. Further studies are required to define the optimal duration of therapy, the necessary components of therapy, and its impact on a wider range of patients.

7. Multidisciplinary team management of stroke patients should be much more widely adopted as a means of ensuring that patients get access to professionals with an interest in stroke.

8. Single-case study designs are an efficient method of testing potentially useful therapies. Treatments that produce benefits should then be evaluated using a conventional randomized controlled trial design.

8 Reducing the risk of recurrent stroke

Clinical trials

To be of use to doctors, information from trials must be generalizable to as many potential patients as possible. This is usually achieved by two means: a large trial, and few restrictions to trial entry. A major problem in many trials of secondary prevention is that they are too small, and if negative run the risk of falsely accepting the null hypothesis (a type II error). Or, in other words, thinking that the difference observed between treated and untreated groups is due to chance. Furthermore, trials should use defined criteria and blind assessment of recurrence to avoid diagnostic and ascertainment bias. Although recurrence rates do not appear to vary with time since onset of the initial stroke, it is sensible to compare recurrence rates over at least one year, and preferably for two to three years. First and subsequent recurrences should be analysed separately to avoid 'double counting' of events. Finally, not all stroke recurrences are equally damaging yet most of the published trials treat them as if they were. An indicator of final disability (such as functional ability, walking, etc.) used as a trial outcome would help clinicians weigh the true benefits of preventing recurrences.

Anti-coagulation after a stroke

At least 13 randomized controlled trials of anti-coagulation after either stroke in evolution or completed stroke had been reported by 1977 (Genton *et al.* 1977). All have been small and suffered from difficulties in precise diagnosis at entry to the trial. In general, subjects had evidence of a stroke but with a clear cerebrospinal fluid (CSF) on lumbar puncture which may not exclude a haemorrhagic stroke. Only one of the studies found any apparent benefit from treatment. This study (Carter 1961) found a reduction in mortality of 55 per cent in patients with progressing stroke but because the numbers were small this apparently impressive difference was not statistically significant. Carter admitted to being uneasy about recommending anti-coagulation because of its risks.

The risks of anti-coagulation were apparent in another UK trial (Hill *et al.* 1962). In an initial study it was found that death and bleeding were much more likely in those with a high (+110 mmHg) diastolic blood pressure. The trial protocol was immediately changed to exclude these subjects and then continued. Patients on active treatment had a higher death rate and 18 per cent of the subjects had an episode of bleeding. There was no difference in recurrent stroke rates.

Table 8.1 shows a summary of 13 trials of 1136 subjects randomized to receive anti-coagulation or no treatment. The pooled odds ratio is 1.11, an 11 per cent treatment benefit. However, the 95 per cent confidence limits are wide (0.8–1.5), indicating the benefit could be as great as 50 per cent or that those on treatment could do up to 20 per cent worse than those not treated. With the added problem of bleeding risks, post-stroke anti-coagulation has never been popular.

It has been claimed that anti-coagulation is of benefit in cerebral embolism. It is argued that because recurrence rates are so high, prophylaxis is necessary (Weksler and Lewin 1983). The evidence for this view includes uncontrolled case series, which tend to give a biased view of treatment benefits, possibly because of publication bias (positive results get published, negative ones often do not). This is analogous to the use of anti-coagulants after myocardial infarction where case series and comparisons with historical controls led to a biased and over-enthusiastic assessment of the effectiveness of anti-coagulation (Chalmers *et al.* 1977; Peto 1978).

Anti-coagulation in stroke and atrial fibrillation

Stroke in the presence of both atrial fibrillation and rheumatic heart disease is an indication, in the eyes of many physicians, to anti-coagulate the patient (Bucknall *et al.* 1986). Starkey and Warlow (1986), in a critical review of the supporting evidence, demonstrated that only one randomized trial had been done and that this was small and showed no advantage of treatment (Baker *et al.* 1962). The evidence of benefit is derived entirely from selected case series, which are no substitute for properly controlled

Table 8.1 Trials of anti-coagulation for secondary stroke prevention taken from Genton *et al.* (1977). Figures are the numbers of subjects in treated and control groups who had no recurrence (success) and a bad outcome (stroke or death: failure). Odds ratios were calculated using Mantel–Haenzel procedure and 95% confidence intervals using Woolf's methods are shown in parentheses

Trial	*Treatment success*	*Control success*	*Treatment failure*	*Control failure*	*Odds of treatment success*
Baker (1961)	20	15	2	0	–
Baker (1962)	18	14	6	6	1.3 (0.3–4.9)
Pearce (1965)	16	15	1	5	5.3 (0.6–51.1)
Baker (1965)	16	21	14	9	0.5 (0.2–1.4)
Carter (1961)	35	31	3	7	2.6 (0.6–11)
Baker (1961)	53	46	8	21	3.0 (1.2–7.5)*
Baker (1962)	60	54	12	6	0.6 (0.2–1.6)
Hill (1962)	44	46	22	19	0.8 (0.4–1.7)
Howard (1963)	12	12	3	3	1.0 (0.2–6)
McDowell (1965)	72	77	20	22	1.0 (0.5–2)
Enger (1965)	46	39	5	10	2.4 (0.7–7.5)

* $P<0.01$, all other odds ratios not significant.

trials. It is now much too late to set up a trial of anti-coagulation of patients with atrial fibrillation and rheumatic heart disease, not only because of established practice but also because of disappearing cases of rheumatic heart disease.

More recently, the issue of anti-coagulation has cropped up again. This time the question is whether anti-coagulants prevent stroke recurrence in patients with a stroke and lone atrial fibrillation. Starkey and Warlow state that: 'it is unsatisfactory and probably unethical as well to treat with anticoagulants patients with stroke and atrial fibrillation but without rheumatic heart disease until we know we are doing more good than harm'.

An opposite Texan view (Sherman *et al.* 1986) concludes that the danger of treatment is worth the risk because of the seriousness of the condition. This unusual reasoning, that ignores the need for treatment to work, is tempered with a call for a randomized controlled trial. Hachinski (1986) thinks that anti-coagulation is justified for a few months, when risks of strokes are high and complications are low but also gives no evidence to support his view. This is the worst sort of advice because it sounds so reasonable, it satisfies the desire to treat, but will depress the impetus to start the necessary trials.

A small non-randomized comparison of a series of 100 stroke patients with non-rheumatic atrial fibrillation treated with anticoagulants in the Netherlands and a series of 50 untreated patients with non-rheumatic atrial fibrillation from the Oxfordshire Community Stroke Project has been published (Lodder *et al.* 1988). Only 70 of the treated patients were included in the analysis because those who had another cardio-embolic source other than lone atrial fibrillation (this was not specified further) or had had a second stroke (presumably before treatment started, although this was not stated) were excluded. The Oxford patients tended to have milder strokes and were older than the Dutch patients. Recurrence rates were similar: 18 per cent among the treated patients and 20 per cent in the Oxford series over a mean follow-up of 27 months. Allowance was made for age and severity and did not affect the findings. The power of the study was acknowledged to be low, and the 95 per cent confidence intervals were compatible with anticoagulation preventing half or leading to a two-fold increase in recurrences and deaths. This study does not contribute much to the debate about the use of anti-coagulants but does indicate that any benefit is likely to be fairly small and a trial of over 1000 patients would be needed to stand a fair chance of detecting a clinically useful benefit. The Dutch investigators have decided to mount such a trial.

Sandercock and colleagues (1986) think that a trial limited to patients with atrial fibrillation is impracticable and irrelevant because only 2 per cent of the patients in the Oxford project would be eligible for such a trial. Moreover, the vast majority of stroke patients in the United Kingdom would never get access to the necessary neuro-radiology to exclude those with intracerebral haemorrhage, thereby ensuring safer use of anti-coagulants (Cerebral Embolism Study Group 1983), and the treatment itself is difficult and expensive to supervise (Stamp *et al.* 1985). The combined results of early work also make it appear to be an unattractive treatment to resurrect.

Risks of anti-coagulation

The risk of bleeding is often given as a reason for not using anti-coagulant treatment, particularly for old people (Roos *et al.* 1965). More recent evidence does not support this view. A Dutch trial of anti-coagulation after myocardial infarction among over 60-year-olds reported a reduction in deaths, recurrent heart attacks and intracranial 'events' in those actively treated, and advanced age was not associated with a greater risk of bleeding (Sixty Plus Reinfarction Study Research Group 1980). Anti-coagulation caused extracranial rather than intracranial bleeding. The chance of a major haemorrhage whilst on treatment was about four bleeds per 100 patient-years of therapy. The background risk of bleeding in the control group was about one bleed per 200 patient-years of observation, and strokes were more common in the control than anti-coagulated group. The excess risk of anti-coagulation was about 2 (95 per cent confidence intervals 0.3–4) major bleeds or strokes per 100 patient-years of treatment. A similar risk of major bleeding was reported by Forfar (1979, 1982), with no excess risk among older people. However, a significant relationship with duration of treatment was found. The risk of bleeding rose from 4 (95 per cent confidence intervals 3–5) per 100 patient-years during the first three years to 14 (95 per cent confidence intervals 8–20) bleeds per 100 patient-years from the fifth to eighth year of follow-up.

The lack of an association between age and risk of bleeding is confirmed by a more recent study (Gurwitz *et al.* 1988).

Anti-coagulation after a stroke would have to prevent more than two recurrences for every 100 patient-years of therapy to ensure a net benefit over its undoubted risks, which may actually be higher in places where very rigorous control, common in Dutch anti-coagulant clinics, is not maintained. This scale of benefit is unlikely since the pooling of studies indicates that anti-coagulation might prevent at best about one stroke or death per 100 patient-years of therapy. However, despite evidence of definite benefit from anti-coagulation after myocardial infarction (Peto 1978), British physicians are distinctly unwilling to use it for this condition (Bucknall *et al.* 1986). A further large trial of anti-coagulation after stroke may also be ignored, whatever its results.

Aspirin

This drug has become a widely but variably used treatment for secondary stroke prevention among both TIA and completed stroke patients (Bucknall *et al.* 1986). Paediatric doses (75 mg tablets), sometimes given alternate days, or 300 mg given weekly, or up to 1.2 g given daily can all be supported from laboratory or clinical trial evidence. Low doses are given in the hope that inhibition of vessel wall prostacyclin will be minimal and of platelet prostaglandin maximal, thus optimizing its anti-thrombotic effects.

At the time most clinical trials were set up, high doses of aspirin were thought to be necessary to achieve effects on platelets, and preliminary results in small series were encouraging. Even the more recent UK–TIA trial compared 1.2 g with 300 mg aspirin and placebo, although it was stated that doses were determined to enable a urine ferric chloride test of compliance with treatment to be used (UK–TIA Study Group 1979; 1988). The study designers should not be criticized for using the 'wrong' dose of aspirin. Trials take a long time to carry out whereas test-tube experiments may advance understanding of pathogenesis very rapidly, apparently making the results of trials of little relevance to up-to-date clinical practice. Clinicians should remember when deciding what to offer patients that the best test of efficacy is obtained by doing trials on people, not extrapolating from studies of isolated vessel walls and platelet suspensions. Laboratory studies are of value in deciding which drugs are worth investigating in human studies, but applying laboratory results to humans directly without trial evidence is most unwise. However, laboratory studies have demonstrated that the 'right' dose of aspirin may be harder to determine than we think. Person-to-person variation in responses to set doses of aspirin are very large; even 1.2 g may not be sufficient to inhibit *in vitro* platelet aggregation in some subjects (Hanley *et al.* 1981; O'Brien 1980), which makes the blanket use of paediatric doses of aspirin even more illogical.

The studies that should help us decide whether to use aspirin have been overviewed (Antiplatelet Trialists' Collaboration 1988). Anti-platelet drugs have been used in 16 trials of patients suffering TIA and stroke. In 13 of the trials aspirin was used, and only five excluded patients with completed stroke. Most of the trials excluded patients with moderate or severe disability. Considerable efforts were made to find all the available published trials, thus avoiding the tendency of reviewers to consider trials that support a particular view.

The overview showed that anti-platelet agents effectively prevented vascular deaths, non-fatal stroke and myocardial infarction among different types of patient with vascular occlusive disease. Low dose aspirin (300 mg daily) was as good as higher doses and other drugs (dipyridamole and sulphinpyrazone), but the results of several very low dose aspirin trials are awaited. Among patients with cerebrovascular disease vascular deaths were reduced by 15 per cent (1–29 per cent), non-fatal strokes by 22 per cent (8–36 per cent), and non-fatal myocardial infarction by 35 per cent (11–59 per cent). Severe strokes were somewhat more likely to be prevented by treatment.

It can be difficult to understand treatment effects if they are expressed as a percentage changes. Sometimes it is not clear if the percentage reported is an absolute difference (i.e. % bad outcomes in controls – % bad outcomes in treated) or a relative difference (i.e. [% bad outcomes in controls – % bad outcomes in treated]/ % bad outcomes in controls). This latter percentage effect is frequently reported as it is usually much greater and therefore more impressive. The relative difference is a more sensible measure to report when comparing trials where event rates in the control group are very different (usually because of differences in selection) because it allows for this variation in the control group event rate.

The method best suited to clinical practice is the number of events prevented per 100 patient-years of treatment which is an absolute difference and dependent on the background recurrence risk of the patients considered. It also gives doctors a way of weighing up the benefits and risks of treatment. For example, The Antiplatelet Trialists' Collaboration calculated the absolute benefits of treatment to be about one fatal and two non-fatal events averted for every 100 patients treated for two years, assuming a fairly low background event rate appropriate for young patients with TIA. Among older patients with completed stroke where the background risk is higher the absolute benefits of treatment will be much larger. If annual vascular event and death rates are both 10 per cent, then aspirin should reduce recurrent stroke to 8 per cent and death to 8.5 per cent, which is equivalent to four non-fatal events and three deaths prevented for every 100 patients treated for two years.

Overviews or meta-analyses are a useful way of trying to decide on the effects of treatments that have only small effects, but because stroke is common may lead to substantial net benefits. A danger of meta-analyses is that only available (usually published) studies can be included, and publication bias—the likelihood that studies showing benefits are more often reported—can lead to a biased assessment of the true effects of a treatment. The effect of this can be demonstrated by using a 'funnel plot' (Vandenbroucke 1988). The odds ratios of treatment effects found in each study are plotted against its sample size (or some proxy measure, such as the standard error of the odds ratio). The scatter of odds ratios around the pooled estimate should be greatest where statistical power is weakest. If publication bias has occurred, weak studies which found no benefit of treatment should be missing from the 'funnel'. The overview published by the Antiplatelet Trialists' Collaboration did not use this technique, but a funnel plot of the data (see Fig. 8.1) did not demonstate any publication bias.

A more obvious danger of a meta-analysis is to conduct it before large trials have been reported. An American meta-analysis was carried out before both the UK–TIA and European studies of aspirin were reported, despite both nearing completion (Sze *et al.* 1988). This analysis found that aspirin compared with placebo was associated with a non-significant 15 per cent reduction in stroke.

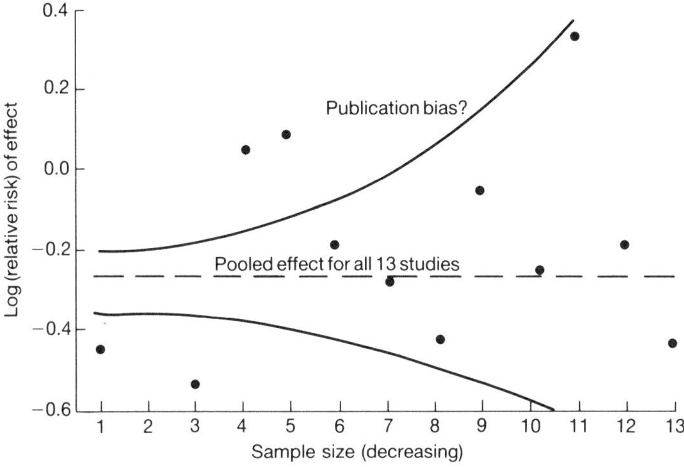

Fig. 8.1 Funnel plot of aspirin in secondary stroke prevention.

Risks of aspirin

The benefits of aspirin treatment must be set against its dangers which can be calculated from some of the trials. The Canadian Cooperative study (1978) recorded one gastro-intestinal bleed during every 100 patient-years of treatment with 1 g daily. In Bousser's *et al.* trial (1983), about two withdrawals from treatment per 100 patient-years of therapy occurred, although a wider range of side-effects was included, which probably explains the higher risk of aspirin observed. The UK–TIA Study (1988) reported severe (i.e. leading to hospital admission) gastro-intestinal bleeding of about 0.4 per cent per year with 300 mg aspirin and 0.6 per cent per year with 1.2 g aspirin, i.e. around one bleed during 200 patient-years of treatment. Looking at these absolute differences helps the clinician get a feel for the amount of prescribing needed to achieve quite small gains. However, these benefits are very similar to those achieved by accepted treatments such as beta-blockade after myocardial infarction or thiazide treatment of moderate hypertension (Antiplatelet Trialists' Collaboration 1988).

The pooled trials show a beneficial effect of aspirin, thus current practice should not change but should be extended to include patients with strokes as well as TIAs. As it is very unlikely that further aspirin studies will be instigated, doctors have to decide how far to apply the results of present work. As event rates in older, more severely affected patients are higher, and absolute benefits of treatment likely to be greater, treating these patients is reasonable. Treating any stroke patient, regardless of severity, who has survived the first month with 300 mg of enteric-coated aspirin daily seems a sensible option. If this leads to gastro-intestinal problems substitution of dipyridamole or sulphinpyrazone can be tried, on the evidence of the studies that have used combinations of antiplatelet agents (Antiplatelet Trialists' Collaboration 1988). The question of how long to continue treatment remains, but since recurrence and death rates do not decrease with time after the stroke, it is probably best to continue indefinitely.

Aspirin does not appear to be effective therapy for women in some of the trials, but this has generally been attributed to chance, or the small number of women studied (Canadian Cooperative Study 1978). However, *in vitro* evidence shows that aspirin exerts greater inhibitory actions on platelet aggregation tests for men than for women (Spranger *et al.* 1989). It will be important in future clinical trials to ensure that data from men and women are analysed separately, and future pooling studies should conduct separate analyses for men and women.

Lowering blood pressure

Randomized trials

Only two randomized trials of the effects of treating high blood pressure after stroke have been published. The first randomized patients under 80 years old suffering a clinically diagnosed ischaemic stroke (Carter 1970). Patients with pressures over 110 mmHg diastolic (phase unmentioned but probably phase IV at this time in the United Kingdom) or a systolic of 160 mmHg or more for over two weeks whilst in hospital were randomized. Forty-nine patients were treated with various anti-hypertensive drugs and 48 were left untreated. The patients were followed-up for four years on average and during this time 44 per cent of the controls and 20 per cent of the treated patients suffered a major or fatal stroke. Deaths from heart failure and myocardial infarction were no different between the groups. The 95 per cent confidence intervals of this 24 per cent difference were 6–42 per cent indicating a significant effect. Patients over the age of 65 did not share this very beneficial effect but numbers were too small to accept or refute the null hypothesis.

The second randomized controlled trial (Hypertension Stroke Cooperative Study Group 1974) was multi-centre, and randomized 452 patients, 80 per cent of whom were Black, and only 9 per cent over the age of 70. Four-fifths had suffered a completed stroke and the remainder a TIA. Although active treatment did lower pressures by about 25 mmHg systolic and 12 mmHg diastolic (from an average of 167/100 [Phase V] at entry), no significant difference in stroke recurrence was observed. The cumulative five year incidence of recurrent stroke was 21 per cent and 24 per cent in the treated and control groups respectively. The 95 per cent confidence limits of this difference are about −5 to 11 per cent, so the study was able to rule out a true treatment effect of more than 11 per cent. However, the observed recurrence rates were very low and suggest that under-reporting of events might have occurred with a bias towards those on therapy (with its side-effects) seeking out their physicians and reporting more events, thus leading to the small observed difference. Furthermore, the blood pressures were probably lower at entry than in Carter's trial (1970), so it is possible that treating milder hypertension after a stroke is not beneficial.

An uncontrolled comparison

An observational study by Beevers and colleagues (1973) is often quoted as evidence of the effectiveness of treating high blood pressures after stroke. The starting point of this study was a clinical series of 162 patients with a past history of both a stroke and hypertension. An imaginary control group was assembled from a review of the literature which comprised data on recurrence of stroke from various series of patients (without regard for blood pressure) and Carter's untreated control patients (1970). Beevers concluded that a recurrence rate of about 40 per cent over four years could be expected. He interpreted the observed recurrence rate of 29 per cent in his series as a favourable effect of therapy when compared with the imaginary control group. Those patients with the best control of their pressures (mean diastolic below 100 mmHg, no phase mentioned) had fewest recurrences (16 per cent), whereas the patients with the worst control (mean diastolic 110 mmHg or more) had the highest risk (55 per cent) of recurrence. It is quite possible that the observed recurrence rates depended as much on selection effects, non-blind counting of events, changing criteria for an event, and different lengths of follow-up as a true effect of treatments.

A common error when analysing observational data is to ignore the effect of duration of follow-up when making comparisons between sub-groups. In clinical trials this may not make too much difference as randomization will ensure that follow-up will be more or less equal between treated and control groups. In Beevers' series the patients with 'poor' control may have been attending the clinic longer than those with 'good' control. Indeed, in routine practice the main reason for attending a hospital clinic is difficulty in reducing blood pressure. Thus, these badly controlled patients may have been around for a longer time than newer well controlled patients. A similar risk of recurrence applied over a longer time will give the impression of higher recurrence among the badly controlled patients if numbers of recurrences are compared. Allowance for length of follow-up must be made and is usually done by using life table methods or patient-years at risk rather than patients as the denominator when calculating rates of recurrence (Peto *et al.* 1976, 1977). In Beevers' study it is impossible to make this allowance because insufficient data were reported. Uncontrolled observations are difficult to interpret even if analysed appropriately and should not be taken at their face value as supporting the case for treatment.

The observations of recurrence and survival among stroke patients in Rochester, Minnesota, US, are interesting because the effects of pre-stroke blood pressure (within one year of the initial stroke) and treatment for high blood pressure during the first year after the initial stroke were related to subsequent events (Meissner *et al.* 1988). Diastolic (but not systolic) pre-stroke blood pressure was related to subsequent mortality, especially in the first three years after the stroke. Treatment aimed at controlling blood pressure after the stroke had no effect on either survival or stroke recurrence over a 10 year period. The authors suggested that the occurrence of a first stroke is such a powerful risk factor for a subsequent stroke it wipes out the potentially modest benefits of treating high blood pressure following a stroke.

Dangers of anti-hypertensive treatment

Sudden lowering of the blood pressure in acute stroke patients may lead to disastrous lack of perfusion of the brain, particularly around the lesion, which may worsen the stroke. Furthermore, it is suggested that lowering the blood pressure too much may precipitate a myocardial infarction (Cruickshank *et al.* 1987). The dangers of lowering blood pressure in the acute phase of a stroke have been documented by case histories (Jansen *et al.* 1986*a*) but not from the two randomized trials in which no evidence of therapy causing strokes or other serious problems was reported (Carter 1970; Hypertension Stroke Cooperative Study Group 1974).

In a study of 100 consecutive hospital admissions for acute stroke or TIA (Jansen *et al.* 1986*b*) a relationship between starting diuretics and the onset of symptoms was found in four cases. Ideally, the authors should have collected a series of control patients admitted to the same hospital but without stroke and documented their therapy over the three weeks prior to admission as they did with their series of stroke patients. This case control method would have given an estimate of the relative risk of suffering a stroke associated with starting anti-hypertensive therapy. The findings as reported do not demonstrate that starting anti-hypertensive drugs is associated with an increased risk of stroke.

Massive falls from admission blood pressures over the first two months were demonstrated by Adams (1965), using blood pressure data from a sub-group of 35 of 729 patients admitted to hospital with acute stroke. The average falls observed were 50 mmHg and 20 mmHg in systolic and diastolic pressures respectively. The reasons for this fall include acute effects of the stroke, regression to the mean (a tendency for very extreme values of a continuously distributed variable to become less extreme with repeated measurement), and adjustment of patients to their environment. The implication for therapy is that repeated measurements are needed to define which patients may need treatment.

The easy way out of the treat or not to treat dilemma is to use the substantial amount of evidence that treatment is effective in primary prevention trials of people who have not yet had a stroke (Veterans Administration 1970; Hypertension Detection and Follow Up Programme 1979; WHO/ISH Mild Hypertension Liaison Committee 1982; Anonymous 1985; Harrison 1984).

Certainly, patients who have had TIAs or mild strokes but have diastolic pressures over 100 mmHg (phase V) should be treated if the wisdom of the MRC and European Working Party on High Blood Pressure in the Elderly trials are followed (MRC Working Party 1985; Amery *et al.* 1985; Amery *et al.* 1986). The questions of how they should be treated, for example with 'new' drugs rather than older, riskier drugs (Wilcox *et al.* 1986), and how far blood pressures should be lowered remain open.

Patients with major strokes and the very old stroke patient are not very typical of subjects recruited into any of the major primary prevention trials and it is therefore difficult to generalize trial results to these groups. Establishing a trial of anti-hypertensives for elderly stroke patients would be problematic. Although recurrence rates are likely to be high in such patients, to detect a 50 per cent relative treatment effect (i.e. an absolute difference of about three recurrences prevented per 100 patient-years of treatment) would require over 1000 patient-years of observation in both the treated and control groups. Such a trial may never be done, so it is sensible to act on the existing evidence and treat any patient with persistently raised blood pressure (over 100 mmHg [phase V], or 160 mmHg systolic) in the non-hemiplegic arm, taken with the patient standing, if possible. Until there is better evidence of the effects of treatment in patients over the age of 80 the best option is to include them in this recommendation, providing that care is taken to monitor adverse side effects. Thiazide diuretics should be used as first line treatment (Amery *et al.* 1985), and because ischaemic heart disease is so common in stroke patients, a case can be made for using beta-blockade as an alternative (Peto 1982).

Carotid endarterectomy

Only two randomized controlled trials to assess the effects of this operation after TIA have been reported (Fields *et al.* 1970; Shaw *et al.* 1984). A high early risk of recurrence following surgery offsetting a later benefit was found. The UK–TIA Study Group (1983) demonstrated that investigation, referral, and operation rates varied dramatically throughout the United Kingdom. The same variation was found in the United States, although the operation rates were about twice as high (Haerer *et al.* 1977). Differences in the type of patient seen did not explain this variation, but the beliefs of physicians and surgeons about the effectiveness of the operation were the most plausible explanation.

Professional practice was examined by asking a panel to rate the appropriateness of indications for carotid endarterectomy, and then these criteria were applied to three geographical sites in the United States during 1981 (Winslow *et al.* 1988). The proportions of appropriate, inappropriate, and equivocal carotid endarterectomies performed at each site were compared, together with outcomes of operation. Overall, 32 per cent of 1302 operations assessed were for equivocal and 32 per cent for inappropriate indications. The main reasons for inapproprate operation were operations for less than 50 per cent stenosis, and operations on patients not suffering carotid distribution transient ischaemic attacks. Moreover, it was surprising that almost a fifth of patients were not being treated with anti-platelet or anti-coagulant therapy, and only 16 (1.2 per cent) of the patients operated on were Black, perhaps implying that economic and social rather than medical criteria were determining use of the operation. Of great concern were the operative risks which were extremely high; 9.8 per cent suffered a major complication (stroke with residual deficit at the time of discharge from hospital or death within 30 days of operation). The authors concluded that carotid endarterectomy was substantially overused, and in the hands of most surgeons, operative risks were too high to lead to any net benefit of the procedure. The authors stated that only patients with appropriate indications should be offered surgery, and that complication rates should be monitored.

However, it has been noted that because many surgeons, especially in the United Kingdom, do fewer than 30 operations a year, it could take from 5 to 15 years before a surgeon with an unacceptable operative risk realized it (Michaels 1988). The operative risk was very high in the UK–TIA series with a quarter suffering a perioperative stroke. It is unacceptable to operate when the annual risk of a stroke is of the order of 10 per cent and the operative risk is more than twice this. It is becoming clearer that the clinical freedom of surgeons to decide on whom they will operate, and the number of operations they will perform is not consistent with good quality practice for patients. Certainly attempts to widen the indications for operation to asymptomatic patients and those with less severe stenosis should be resisted because of their low risk of stroke.

As the operation may have a long-term protective effect (Fields *et al.* 1970), it has been argued that if peri-operative risks were lower the operation would be useful. A threshold of 5 per cent for operative risks of stroke and/or death has been recommended as acceptable in the face of a stroke rate of about 10 per cent a year (UK–TIA Study Group 1983). However, the recent trials of aspirin after TIA and mild stroke have demonstrated lower attack rates—about 6 per cent a year (Antiplatelet Trialists' Collaboration 1988), which may be reduced further by use of aspirin and anti-hypertensives. This makes carotid endarterectomy useless unless operative risks can be reduced to below 2 to 3 per cent. Most centres in the United Kingdom will never do enough operations to achieve such a figure, so the operation's future lies in centralization with highly experienced surgeons, probably doing little else. An Anglo-French randomized controlled trial has been started to re-examine the effectiveness of the operation for patients with carotid territory TIAs or mild strokes, and may clarify its future.

Extracranial-intracranial bypass surgery

There is potential for conflict between trialists and clinicians. The heated discussion in the *British Medical Journal* caused by a trial of extracranial bypass surgery for stroke patients (EC/IC Bypass Study Group 1985) illustrated some of the misunderstandings between trialists and clinicians.

Anastomosis of the superficial temporal artery to the middle cerebral artery (EC/IC bypass) has been described as: 'an elegant procedure without a clinical indication' (Wade 1987). The Canadian initiated international randomized controlled trial of EC/IC bypass was set up in 1977 to measure the rates of stroke recurrence in a group treated with this novel operation and a control group treated medically. The trial randomized 1377 patients: 714 to medical treatment and 663 to surgery and followed them up for 56 months, on average. The patients were young (mean age 56 years), four-fifths were men, and over 90 per cent had minimal or no functional impairment. A third had only had a TIA but many had other problems: half were hypertensive, nearly a fifth had diabetes and 10 per cent had a previous myocardial infarction. Both groups were actively treated with aspirin (75 per cent of patients) and anti-hypertensives.

Surgery did not reduce the risk of recurrence despite being competently performed (96 per cent of anastomoses were patent at final angiographic review). During the perio-operative period, stroke occurred in more than three out of every 100 operations. By the end of the study the cumulative risk of stroke recurrence was about 30 per cent in both groups. There were no differences in death rates or functional disability either. The results might have occurred by chance but the probability of accepting the null hypothesis of no benefit when in fact a benefit existed (i.e. a type II error) was less than 1 in 100. The trial was designed and carried out in an exemplary way: it was large, the follow-up was long, patient groups were fairly homogeneous, and well balanced, there were no follow-up losses, event criteria were applied by 'blind' adjudicators, similar 'background' therapy was used between both groups and the surgical technique was effective.

The recurrence rate reported in the EC/IC trial was similar to other less selected series, although with the supposed benefits of modern medical therapy (aspirin and anti-hypertensives) they might have been expected to do rather better. The trial patients were comparatively young, had minimal or no obvious impairments at randomization, but most had other evidence of arterial disease. These facts help in deciding to whom *not* to recommend surgery. It is this very group who are most at risk of well-intentioned but possibly harmful effects of this operation.

One weakness of the study was in documenting what happened to non-randomized but eligible patients. This led to a contentious article (Dudley 1987) suggesting that the trial results could not be generalized because: 'The trial was biased' due to the exclusion of possibly one-half to three-quarters of eligible patients. 'Biased' and 'partial' randomization were referred to which are worrying concepts implying that the method of randomization was at fault, permitting patients to enter the control or treatment group in a non-random way. This would, of course, seriously affect the validity of the trial. The main criticism of the trial was not its validity (which was not in serious doubt) but the question of its generalizability to other settings. Professors Warlow and Peto (1987) considered this question and pointed out that the trial applied to patients who were: 'reasonably similar' to those randomized. There is no scientific way of determining what this means but common sense and judgement should be used. Baum (1987) highlighted the 'Catch 22' of generalizability and validity. Having accepted that a trial has given a valid result which is disliked, the last-ditch stand to take in refuting its results is to claim it lacks generalizability. This ruse permits clinicians to continue backing their hunches and pursuing their freedom to go on offering the treatment. Such an approach defies both common sense and medical judgement.

Summary

1. Specific treatments that should be offered to patients with TIAs or strokes (any severity) are aspirin in moderate dose (300 mg daily), and anti-hypertensives to those with systolic pressures over 160 mmHg or diastolic phase V pressures above 100 mmHg.

2. Anti-coagulation after a stroke is not associated with any net benefit but there is insufficient evidence to make a clear assessment. The risks of treatment appear to outweigh possible benefits of treatment on present evidence. If anti-coagulation is used, CT scanning should be done before starting anti-coagulation to exclude cases of haemorrhagic stroke.

3. Carotid endarterectomy surgery is too dangerous to be of benefit in the United Kingdom and United States, and is over-used in the latter. Extracranial-intracranial bypass surgery is not effective.

4. Information on final level of ability and quality of life is badly needed to complement recurrence rates as outcome measures in trials, together with an economic appraisal of treatment effects (e.g. days spent in hospital, use of community services).

Part III

Prognosis

9 Mortality after stroke

Why should doctors bother to understand the pattern and predictors of death after a stroke? Knowing when death is most likely and what causes it should help decide where to concentrate effort and lead to innovations in treatment. Perhaps the devastating nature of some strokes leads doctors to feel that death is not a bad outcome, and indeed preferable to a lengthy period of rehabilitation leading to a long-stay hospital bed. This gloomy outlook is far from the truth for the majority of patients (see Chapter 12, on recovery). Information about prognosis is useful for the following reasons:

(1) patients and relatives need information to plan their lives;
(2) to permit triage of patients with different prognosis, thus allowing rationing of resources and balanced comparisons in treatment trials;
(3) to identify patients with a poor prognosis who may benefit from special efforts;
(4) to find predictors of poor prognosis that may be amenable to change, and thus possibly improve prognosis.

Risk of dying

The risk of dying after a stroke has been widely studied but perhaps the most surprising fact is how variable reported case fatality rates are, ranging from 7 to 67 per cent dead by one year (Marshall and Shaw 1959; Stevens and Ambler 1982). The most obvious explanation is that selection bias is responsible for much of the variation. However, even when a standardized protocol was used in a WHO multi-centre study, almost two-fold variation in one year case fatality rates occurred between participating centres (Aho *et al.* 1980), see Table 9.1.

The variation in case fatality is as marked between hospital series as community series. This is because the studies also differed in age composition, which together with differences in ascertainment of cases of stroke, have a marked effect on subsequent mortality. In

Table 9.1 Variation in cumulative mortality in hospital and community series of stroke patients

Source	*Time since stroke (%)*			
	One week	*Three weeks*	*Three months*	*One year*
Community patients				
Aho *et al.* (1980)	25	33	40	50
Bonita *et al.* (1984)	23	34[a]		48
Eisenberg *et al.* (1964)		56		85[d]
Harmsen and Wilhelmsen (1984)	22	27		36
Herman *et al.* (1980)	19	26		
Sacco *et al.* (1982)		22[a]		35[c]
Stevens and Ambler (1982)		45[a]		67
Wade and Hewer (1987)			34[b]	
Weddell and Beresford (1979)	34	45	54	80[c]
Hospital patients				
Adams and Merrett (1961)				20
Barer (1987)		32[a]	46[b]	
Carter (1964)				37
Droller (1960)				24
Henley *et al.* (1985)			30[b]	44
Kotila *et al.* (1984)			35	40
Marshall and Shaw (1959)				7
Marquardsen (1969)	35	46		59
Sheikh *et al.* (1983)		28		49
Schmidt *et al.* (1988)		37		72[d]

[a] 1 month; [b] 6 months; [c] 4 years; [d] 5 years.

Weddell and Beresford's study (1979), every effort was made to register cases occurring in a defined population and many cases were derived from death certificates which almost certainly accounts for the high one week case fatality rate reported. In Herman *et al.*'s study (1980), patients had to be seen by a doctor before registration, which may account for the rather low case fatality, because early deaths were not registered.

It is probable that patients admitted to hospital have worse strokes and a worse survival. In Weddell's study three week case fatality among men, but not women, was three times higher in those admitted to hospital (75 per cent died). In the Oxfordshire Community Stroke Project patients with impaired consciousness were almost four times more likely to be admitted to hospital (Bamford *et al.* 1986), which should lead to improved overall case fatality of those kept at home due to selective admission of those with the worst prognosis.

Longer-term survival of stroke patients is much worse than in the general population. Annual risks of dying of about 10 per cent for stroke patients under 60 years, 15 per cent at ages 60–69, 25 per cent at ages 70–79, and 50 per cent for those over 80 years were reported by Marquardsen (1969). These rates are about 18–24 times expected rates in the general population for those under 60, and about twice expected rates for those over 70 years.

The only consistent finding in these studies is that the majority of deaths occur within the first three weeks, further deaths occur over the first year, and then deaths continue at a constant age-dependent but increased rate compared with the general population.

Causes of death after stroke

Even if every patient had a post-mortem examination it would be impossible to resolve the 'what did this patient die from?' and the 'what did this patient die with?' dilemma. The findings at necropsy in a small hospital series where virtually all early deaths were examined were: brain swelling; pulmonary emboli; and recent myocardial infarction (Oxbury *et al.* 1975). When hospital patients were followed up for six months, the percentage of deaths attributed to each cause was as follows: primary brain death (16 per cent); pneumonia (44 per cent); pulmonary embolism (25 per cent); heart failure, myocardial infarction or arrhythmia (12 per cent); renal failure (2 per cent); other causes (2 per cent) (Barer 1987). Follow-up to death gives a different picture: recurrent stroke (23 per cent); myocardial infarction (10 per cent); heart failure and/or bronchopneumonia (30 per cent); pulmonary infarction (5 per cent); uraemia (3 per cent) (Marquardsen 1969). The preponderance of ischaemic heart disease deaths during the later phases of follow-up is confirmed by other studies, and appears to continue for several years (Viitanen *et al.* 1987; Scmidt *et al.* 1988).

Predictors of early mortality

Conscious level

Predictors of early mortality after stroke noted over 100 years ago were impaired conscious level, breathing abnormalities, bilateral neurological signs, and hypothermia followed by pyrexia (Marquardsen 1969). Impaired consciousness has stood the test of time as an adverse prognostic sign for survival. In the WHO stroke registration project (Aho *et al.* 1980) three week case fatality was 15 times higher in comatose compared with alert patients. The strength of this association varies from four- to five-fold in most studies (Rankin 1957; Marquardsen 1969; Oxbury *et al.* 1975) falling as low as just over two-fold in one retrospective hospital series (Lowe *et al.* 1983). Most studies have found a stepwise gradient of risk of death with increasing level of unconsciousness. However, a few initially comatose stroke patients do eventually make a good recovery.

Type of stroke

Although early studies were not able to diagnose type of pathology adequately, most studies have reported very high case fatality for haemorrhagic stroke; from seven-fold increased first day mortality (Marquardsen 1969), to two-fold increased one month mortality (Eisenberg 1964; Harmsen and Wilhemsen 1984; Herman *et al.* 1982*a*; Garraway *et al.* 1983*a*; Sacco *et al.* 1982).

The major problem with clinical diagnosis of cerebral haemorrhage is that an adverse prognostic variable—unconsciousness—is part of the criteria for diagnosing haemorrhagic stroke (see, for example, Tanaka *et al.* 1981), which confounds the relationship between pathology and mortality. Neuro-radiology is required to permit accurate diagnosis and avoid linking unconsciousness, a prognostic indicator, with the means of making the diagnosis. The Oxfordshire Community Stroke Project was able to make a neuroradiological diagnosis in a very high proportion of patients and found a four-fold higher case fatality in haemorrhagic stroke than ischaemic stroke (J. Bamford, MD dissertation). This difference is very similar to clinically diagnosed Framingham patients where 30 day mortality was 82 per cent for haemorrhagic and 15 per cent for thrombotic stroke (Sacco *et al.* 1982).

Although clinical diagnostic criteria are too inaccurate to classify individual patients, they appear sufficiently accurate to compare survival in groups of patients, especially if standardized assessments are made (Sandercock *et al.* 1985*a*). Ideally, the impact of possible predictors of case fatality should be examined separately for ischaemic, haemorrhagic, and lacunar stroke but this information is not yet available. In practice, mortality after the first few weeks is likely to be among patients with ischaemic stroke, whereas haemorrhagic stroke will tend to weight the early mortality.

Other predictors

Predictors of early mortality (within the first three weeks) include high blood pressure on admission to hospital (Aho *et al.* 1980; Marquardsen 1969; Rankin 1957), age (Marquardsen 1969; Herman *et al.* 1982*a*; Sacco *et al.* 1982), raised blood glucose (Power *et al.* 1988) raised haematocrit and atrial fibrillation (Lowe *et al.* 1983; Sandercock *et al.* 1986), pupil changes, gaze paresis, extensor plantar responses, abnormal breathing, abnormal body temperature, and meningeal irritation (Rankin 1957; Marquardsen 1969), and dysphagia (Barer 1987, 1989; Gordon *et al.* 1987). Table 9.2 lists predictors of early (within one month) and late mortality, together with an indication of how strongly they are associated with mortality.

Some of the predictors listed in Table 9.2 tend to be associated with each other as well as with mortality. Combinations of predictors that predict survival and death more accurately have been sought. Any combination of unconsciousness, gaze paresis, and dense hemiplegia was said to be a better predictor of early death in a series of patients with clinically diagnosed cerebral thrombosis (Oxbury *et al.* 1975). As is shown in Table 9.3, adding gaze paresis and dense hemiplegia to conscious level actually reduces the accuracy of the prediction of death compared with using conscious level alone.

Another attempt to produce an overall score (level of consciousness, orientation, speech, gaze paresis, facial weakness, motor strength, disability, spasticity, and sensation) achieved higher predictive accuracy, around 66 per cent, but this was only slightly better than the 50 per cent accuracy of subjective predictions made by the admitting doctor (Britton *et al.* 1980*a*).

Sheikh and colleagues (1983) have tried to unravel the independent contributions of several prognostic variables using multiple regression. Impaired consciousness, conjugate deviation of eyes,

Table 9.2 Relative risk estimates of the strength of association of predictors with early and late mortality after stroke

Factor	*Early mortality*	*Late mortality*
Alert vs. not alert	2.3–15	2.6–4
Haemorrhagic vs. thrombotic stroke	2–5.5	
Dysphagia	5	3.6
Pupil abnormality	1.6–3	
Gaze paresis	1.8	
Extensor planters	2.2–2.6	
Pyrexia	1.9	
Abnormal breathing	2.2–2.9	
Haematocrit 50% +	2	
Blood glucose >7 mmol/l		3.8
Meningeal irritation	1.4	
Barthel <5 out of 20		4.5
Incontinence of urine		4–5
Blood pressure (+240 mmHg)	2	4
Pre-stroke hypertension		2–5
Heart disease/hypertension		3–5
Age over 70	2	2
Atrial fibrillation	1.3–3	1
Past stroke		2

Table 9.3 Predictive accuracy of conscious level, gaze paresis, and dense hemiplegia for early mortality after stroke (from Oxbury *et al.* 1975)

Factor	*Dead*	*Alive*	*Factor*	*Dead*	*Alive*
Not alert	15	26	Any present	15	38
Alert	0	52	None present	0	40
Predictive value for death	15/(15+26) (37%)		Predictive value for death	15/(15+38) (28%)	

age, and severity of motor deficit correctly predicted 73 per cent of deaths within the first three weeks. The effects of a history of heart disease, previous stroke, and pupil abnormalities were not important. However, haematocrit, heart rhythm, temperature, and blood pressure, among other known predictors of death, were not included in the multivariate model.

Predictors of late mortality

Mortality beyond six months is probably increased by pre-stroke high blood pressure (Sacco *et al.* 1982), although blood pressure measured after the stroke does not predict mortality (Merrett and Adams 1966). Age remains a good predictor of late mortality (Marquardsen 1969; Aho *et al.* 1980; Bonita *et al.* 1984), together with indicators of severity of stroke (Wylie 1962; Aho *et al.* 1980; Marquardsen 1969) and past history of stroke (Aho *et al.* 1980; Bonita *et al.* 1984). Conscious level probably continues to have some predictive effect even one year after the stroke (Christie 1981). The strength of these associations is shown in Table 9.2.

Multiple regression has been used to predict late mortality. Level of consciousness, age, combined neurological deficits, sensory deficit, and gaze paresis each contributed independently to improving the prediction at one year (Sheikh *et al.* 1983).

Activities of daily living

In a selected group of patients receiving rehabilitation and followed for two years, a score comprising age, walking ability, a past history of myocardial infarction (both measured at variable times up to three months after the stroke) predicted 74 per cent of deaths and 79 per cent of survivors (Wade *et al.* 1984*a*). In a community series of patients poor activities of daily living alone (Barthel score less than 5 out of 20 during the first week) gave similar accuracy, correctly predicting 67 per cent of six month deaths and 85 per cent of survivors (Wade and Hewer 1987). The powerful predictive effect of activities of daily living scores on subsequent mortality has also been shown by others (Wylie 1967; Ebrahim *et al.* 1985*b*).

Urinary incontinence

Urinary incontinence in the first week of a stroke is claimed to be a better predictor than conscious level of late mortality (Wade and

Hewer 1985*a*). Six month mortality was predicted by urinary incontinence in 60 per cent of cases, which was no better than prediction using loss of consciousness at onset of the stroke. The predictive value of both incontinence and loss of consciousness is shown in Table 9.4.

Triage

As conscious level makes such a large impact on both early and late survival prospects, swamping the contribution of other predictors, other measures of stroke severity (gaze paresis, sensory and motor deficit, etc.) it is of great use in triage of patients for specialist rehabilitation. Conscious level is also much easier to measure than many predictors. It has been used successfully with walking ability and pre-stroke disability to allocate patients to a stroke unit (Garraway *et al.* 1981). Refining severity factors into an overall score is not worthwhile as a more complicated system for deciding on place of treatment would be time consuming and difficult to standardize. Prognostic indicators are not sufficiently accurate to be used to decide whether or not to with hold supportive treatment in the acute phase (Barer and Mitchell 1989).

Modifying predictors

It is disappointing that factors which reflect stroke severity continue

Table 9.4 Accuracy of predicting death and survival at six months comparing urinary incontinence and loss of consciousness (from Wade and Hewer 1985)

Consciousness	*Dead*	*Alive*	*Urinary incontinence*	*Dead*	*Alive*
Lost	94	60	Present	138	92
Not lost	84	281	Absent	42	251
Predictive value for death	94/(94 + 60) (61%)		Predictive value for death	138/(138 + 92) (60%)	
Predictive value for survival	281/(84 + 281) (77%)		Predictive value for survival	251/(42 + 251) (86%)	

to have such a large effect because this implies that improved late survival may only be achieved by reducing the initial severity of the stroke.

Of predictors and causes of late mortality, a history of hypertension and heart disease suggest that treatment of these problems may lead to improved survival. Treating hypertension after a stroke may be beneficial (see Chapter 8 on reducing the risks of recurrent stroke) and treating moderate to severe heart failure improves survival in other groups (Anonymous 1987*a*). Prevention of deep vein thrombosis and pulmonary emboli by subcutaneous heparin may produce a small improvement in survival (McCarthy and Turner 1986), although the risks of precipitating an intracerebral bleed need to be precisely measured in larger trials. Urinary incontinence and poor activities of daily living may be simply markers of stroke severity and hence little may be done to modify them.

However, case fatality among rehabilitation, acute hospital, and community patients has fallen over the last 40 years (Hurwitz and Adams 1972; Haberman *et al.* 1978; Garraway *et al.* 1983*a*). These trends may be due to the effects of increased ascertainment of milder strokes, treatment of coexisting disease, avoidance of disability through rehabilitation, an increased 'biological fitness' of patients now suffering stroke, changes in the proportion of haemorrhagic to thrombo-embolic strokes, improvements in the environment, such as central heating, and better social support. It is possible that some of the adverse prognosis of age may be mediated through such factors, and indeed the influence of age on functional recovery is not strong (see Chapter 12 on recovery).

More attention should be given to looking for predictors of early and late mortality that are independent of stroke severity or conscious level. For example, dysphagia among alert stroke patients on the first day is associated with a four-fold increased risk of death in the first month (Barer 1987). It is possible that dysphagia merely reflects stroke severity, but among alert patients it is equally possible that preventable complications (such as aspiration and dehydration) lead to death.

Summary

1. Between a quarter and a half of deaths occur in the first three weeks after a stroke, and between a third and two-thirds by one

year. After the first year death rates are about twice those expected in the general population for patients over the age of 70 but very much higher than this for younger patients.

2. Level of consciousness on admission is the single best predictor of early death. Only marginal improvements can be made by including other predictors. Better prediction may be achieved by examining survival in pathologically defined groups, as haemorrhagic stroke has such a high early case fatality.

3. Hypertension, heart disease, pneumonia, and pulmonary emboli are important treatable causes of death. Prevention, active detection, and treatment are needed.

4. Triage for rehabilitation (and randomization for acute treatment trials) should use conscious level as the simplest and most discriminating predictor of outcome.

5. Late mortality is still influenced by level of consciousness at onset, but potentially modifiable predictors (independent of stroke severity) such as dysphagia, poor activities of daily living, and urinary incontinence require further study.

10 Recurrent stroke

'Will it happen again, Doctor?' The stroke patient is asking one of the most difficult questions to answer clearly and is expecting a straight yes or no. The clinician may toss a mental coin, and say 'no', realizing that this answer will be wrong some of the time but right most of the time. The response may be justified by the paternalistic notion that the patient really does not need negative ideas to ponder during the difficult period of recovery. An alternative is to give a probability of a further stroke. Depending on the optimism of the doctor this may be stated as a percentage chance of having a stroke or a much bigger chance of not having a stroke. The figure usually quoted is around 10 per cent per year (Allen 1984*a*; Wade *et al.* 1985*b*). However, this leads to a series of questions: a 10 per cent chance of what and for how long? To which of the diseases that comprise stroke does this figure apply? Does it mean the same sort of risk for all sorts of people—men and women, old and young, severely and mildly affected?

The clinician should be able to give a specific answer that helps both himself and the patient to weigh a risk of further stroke against possible preventive treatments (with their own potential risks), rehabilitation efforts, social, and family affairs.

The chances of a recurrent stroke

Marquardsen's early retrospective study (1969) of 769 patients admitted to hospital from 1940 to 1952 is a most important natural history study as it followed-up patients for up to 23 years and gave great detail about recurrence of stroke. The criteria used to define stroke recurrence were 'a definite worsening of the neurological sequelae from the primary stroke, if occurring abruptly'. Events were recorded not as they occurred, but retrospectively, during home visits by Marquardsen himself. This had the virtue that no variation between observers could have occurred, but a single investigator could have changed his rules over such a long time period, and the patients' memories for events might be unreliable.

He found that risk of further stroke (including all subsequent strokes) was 8.9 events per 100 patient-years for men, and 10.6 events per 100 patient-years for women. This risk did not decline as time passed but was higher amongst people aged over 80 (Fig. 10.1).

The cumulative risk of recurrence over five years is high, ranging from about a third to almost a half affected. The background risk of having a stroke, allowing for age, is also shown in Fig. 10.1, using the Oxfordshire Community Stroke Project (1983) incidence rates. A patient over 75 years old, for example, has a risk of stroke of between 1.2 and 1.9 per cent per year. This is equivalent to a cumulative five-year risk of between 6 and 9 per cent. A patient who has suffered a first stroke has a five-year risk of further strokes of 30 to 50 per cent, about four times the general population risk.

The Framingham Study has collected data on stroke recurrence among 394 patients suffering first strokes from 1949 to 1975 in a defined population but found no increased risk with age (Sacco *et al.* 1982). Men had about twice the risk of recurrence of women, with a male five-year cumulative risk of recurrence of 42 per cent

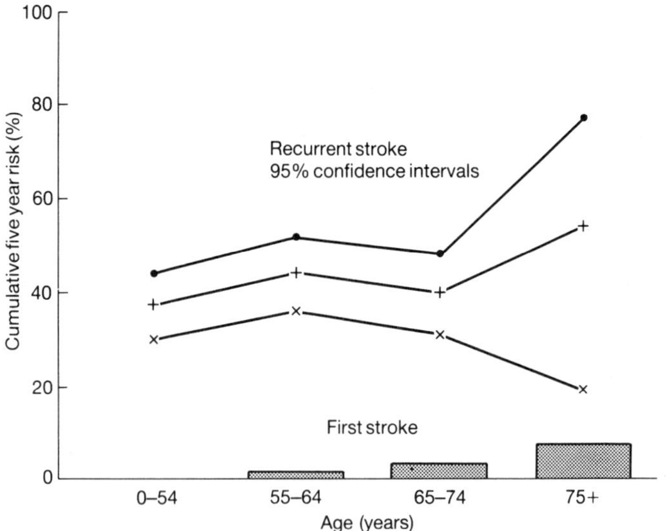

Fig. 10.1 Cumulative risk of recurrent stroke and first stroke after five years.

(an annual risk of about 9 per cent), which is very similar to Marquardsen's hospital series. Women had a five-year risk of 24 per cent, equivalent to an annual risk of 5 per cent. The better prognosis of women is unexplained but was thought to be due to their higher compliance with treatment. It is possible that Marquardsen's higher female risk of recurrence resulted from women admitted to hospital being older, and having more heart disease. Recurrence rates from Rochester, Minnesota, US, were of the same order; 10 per cent in the first year but tended to fall over the next four years to about 4 per cent a year (Whisnant *et al.* 1971; Matsumoto *et al.* 1973). Other studies have not found a decline in recurrence rates after the first year but it could be explained by higher mortality (from both stroke and ischaemic heart disease) among those at highest risk of recurrence, leading to a somewhat 'fitter' survivor group.

Further observation of stroke patients in Rochester, Minnesota, US, from 1950 to 1979 has demonstrated a low recurrence rate of less than 5 per cent per year, with a five-year recurrence rate of 19.3 per cent. Recurrence rates have not changed much over this 30-year time span (Meissner *et al.* 1988). This suggests that the increased use of anti-hypertensives and anti-platelet drugs has either not been sufficiently widely applied, or is of marginal effectiveness compared with the greatly increased risk of recurrent stroke among first stroke survivors.

Blood pressure

Marquardsen highlighted the very poor prognosis of patients with high diastolic blood pressure at the time of the original stroke. Men with diastolic pressures over 120 mmHg (phase and arm used were not reported) on admission had a 4.7-fold increased risk, and women a two-fold risk, of further stroke compared with those with diastolic pressures below 99 mmHg. These blood pressure readings were taken on admission and will tend to be higher than pressures taken a few weeks after the stroke (Adams 1965).

Merrett and Adams (1966) found that patients with high blood pressures (taken several weeks after the stroke, and in older patients referred for rehabilitation) were more, rather than less likely to survive, but they did not measure recurrences. The prognostic importance of blood pressure in older stroke survivors remains a puzzle that needs to be clarified in a population study, using pressures measured at various times, thus avoiding selection and measurement bias.

Johnston and colleagues (1981) using a group of stroke patients attending a blood pressure clinic found higher first visit blood pressures among those suffering a recurrence. The lowest recorded systolic pressure during following up was 20 mmHg lower in the group without a recurrent stroke. This study appears to support the notion that high blood pressure is associated with recurrent stroke but it is quite possible that those with higher pressures stayed under follow-up for longer and thus had more time to suffer another stroke. Incidence rates for recurrent stroke using patient-years of follow-up as a denominator, categorized by level of blood pressure and treatment, should have been calculated so that the risk of recurrent stroke could have been compared in each group.

Type of stroke

Because of the difficulty in diagnosing the pathological process causing a stroke, no separate risk factors were defined for thrombotic, haemorrhagic, or embolic stroke in Marquardsen's study. The recurrence rate for patients suffering transient ischaemic attacks (TIA) and very mild strokes is probably lower than after more severe strokes, about 4 per cent per year in a community series (Heyman *et al.* 1984). An attempt to follow-up a diagnostically 'clean' group of patients with occlusion of the middle cerebral artery suffered from the effects of marked selection (Sacquegna *et al.* 1984). Seventy patients with an average age of 55 years, who had had cerebral angiography between 1970 and 1980 were studied at an Italian Neurology Institute. A cumulative incidence of recurrent stroke of 10.4 per cent at five years, and an annual risk of recurrence of 2 per cent were found. It is likely this estimate is too low for two reasons. First, any group of tertiary referral patients is highly atypical. They survived long enough to be investigated and may therefore be less severely affected than more typical cases. Secondly, the method of counting recurrent strokes by interview or telephoning the family doctor was of doubtful accuracy and might underestimate recurrences.

It has been noted that the survival prospects after cerebral haemorrhage are so poor that any study of recurrence is almost the same as a study of recurrence after cerebral infarction (Sacco *et al.* 1982). Although there is something to be said for this view, in most cases doctors simply do not know which pathological process is taking place, and it is more honest to lump them together under the label of 'stroke'. Until a large population series of neuro-radiologically diagnosed stroke patients is reported, the best estimates of the true recurrence rates among thrombotic, haemorrhagic, and embolic strokes will remain the pooled estimates for all stroke patients. However, if more stroke patients are investigated with CT scans, we may be able to give a more specific prognosis.

Atrial fibrillation

A study of stroke recurrence (Sage and Van Uitert 1983) among 59 patients with atrial fibrillation but no evidence of valve disease reported a recurrence rate of 20 per cent per year, equivalent to a 67 per cent chance of a further stroke over five years. This is about twice the rate expected and compares with Marquardsen's finding of a 1.6- to 1.8-fold increased risk among men and women with atrial fibrillation.

Including early recurrent stroke deaths in figures for recurrent stroke (usual practice) tends to overemphasize the prognostic importance of factors which have their major impact early on, and often lead to death rather than disability. Such factors may not be as relevant to the prognosis of survivors of the early phase. Data from 30-day survivors in the Oxfordshire Community Stroke Project (Sandercock *et al.* 1986) have been analysed separately. Among 30-day survivors there was no impact of atrial fibrillation on subsequent risk of recurrent stroke over the following two years. The recurrence rate among 30-day survivors with and without atrial fibrillation was about 13 per cent within two years. This is lower than the figures obtained by Marquardsen which may be because of the exclusion of early recurrent stroke deaths, the wider community coverage in the Oxford study, the method of counting recurrences and perhaps even the effect of modern medical treatment.

A further factor is that there has been a decline in both mortality and incidence of stroke, which probably started in the United States in the 1940s (Garraway *et al.* 1979; Kotilla 1984*b*). The explanations for this trend are not clear, and it may not be universal; in Sweden a decline in incidence was not found (Alfredsson *et al.*

1986). The effects of treatment (Tuomilehto *et al.* 1985), and improvements in physique and maternal health (Barker and Osmond 1987) are possible explanations for the decline. This latter suggestion is derived from observations that stroke mortality rates parallel falls in maternal mortality in the United Kingdom, and that regions with high maternal mortality were associated with high stroke mortality rates. The pathogenesis of the associations remains obscure. (See Chapter 1 on risk and risk factors).

Other factors

Primary polycythaemia certainly increases the risk of strokes (Pearson and Wetherley-Mein 1978). Whether secondary polycythaemia is associated with an increased risk of recurrent stroke is debatable and the effectiveness of treating such patients is currently under study (Wetherly-Mein *et al.* 1987). Advice to stop smoking (a cause of polycythaemia) in these and other patients can be justified for other reasons despite a lack of evidence that it will reduce recurrence.

Heart failure apparently increases male, but not female, risk of recurrence by 2.6 times (Marquardsen 1969). The Framingham male recurrence rates (Sacco *et al.* 1982) were also greatly increased by the presence of 'cardiac comorbidity'—which meant high blood pressure, heart failure, and coronary heart disease. Male five-year recurrence rates fell from 45 to 28 per cent after removing patients with pre-stroke heart disease and hypertension from analysis. Comparable five-year female recurrence rates only fell from 24 to 19 per cent, with most of this fall due to the effect of hypertension.

The highest recurrence rate found by Marquardsen was 53 per cent per year was among patients with both atrial fibrillation and an average diastolic blood pressure of +100 mmHg (a five-fold increased risk). This suggests that risk factors for recurrent stroke are likely to be multiplicative when their combined effects are assessed. For example, a man with a diastolic blood pressure of over 120 mmHg on admission, atrial fibrillation and heart failure will have a $4.7 \times 2.6 \times 1.6 = 11.7$-fold increased risk of a recurrent stroke.

One of the great strengths of the Framingham data is that all the blood pressures and assessments of heart disease were made before the onset of a stroke. Therefore it is very unlikely that any bias occurred in defining risk factors for recurrence. Selection effects are also less likely as the study was of a community rather than of a hospital-based population.

Summary

1. The overall chance of having a further stroke is about 10 per 100 patient-years, falling to about six per 100 patient-years after surviving the first month. Over the next few years the rate is constant but women have fewer strokes than men. The risk of a completed stroke after a TIA is lower, about 4 per 100 patient-years.

2. The main factors known to increase the risk of a recurrent stroke are male sex, raised blood pressure (before and after the stroke), atrial fibrillation, coexisting ischaemic heart disease, and age over 80 years. These factors increase risk of recurrence by between 1.5 and 2.5 times. Polycythaemia and type of stroke may influence recurrence rates but information is lacking.

11 Effects of stroke

Many of the effects of stroke are not obvious for weeks or months, and by this time the patient is often back at home if admission was sought during the acute phase. Follow-up by rehabilitation teams, hospital, and family doctors after a stroke is patchy, and certainly not related to need—if impairments and disability are accepted as indicators of need (Ebrahim *et al.* 1987*b*), so it is likely that many complications may go undetected. Avoidable complications of stroke have been reviewed (Mulley 1982), and for painful hemiplegic shoulders, spasticity, contractures, constipation, falls, and fractures there is nothing new to add. In the areas of depressed mood, cognition, dysphasia, urinary incontinence, dysphagia, deep vein thrombosis and pulmonary embolism, quality of life, and support for carers, more recent studies are available. The extent of these specific complications, their importance and management will be considered next.

Mood change

Depressed mood has long been known to occur after a stroke (Bleuler 1924) and is of concern, not just because of the human misery involved, but also because it may be a barrier to successful rehabilitation (Adams and Hurwitz 1963). It has been demonstrated that among patients with a relatively good spontaneous recovery, depressed mood is associated with a longer hospital stay, although the importance of depression as a barrier to recovery in more severe strokes is doubtful (Ebrahim *et al.* 1987*a*).

Measurement of the frequency of mood disorder after stroke is beset with problems, particularly of case definition (House 1987). Attempts to use the dexamethasone suppression test as a biological marker of depressed mood have shown that it lacks validity when compared with psychiatric interview (Lipsey *et al.* 1985). Mood rating scales are no substitute for a careful psychiatric interview but may give some indication of the scale of the problem. The General Health Questionnaire (GHQ) is a widely used self-filled questionnaire of affective problems and has been used to measure mood in patients with physical illness (MacGuire *et al.* 1974; Knights and Folstein 1977; Glass *et al.* 1978; Hawton 1981), and after stroke (Robinson and Price 1982; Ebrahim *et al.* 1987*a*). As seven out of 28 GHQ questions are to do with physical difficulty in carrying out daily tasks, many physically ill people will respond positively to them, thus appearing to be depressed. The usual threshold to distinguish those with a high chance of depression from the rest is five or more out of 28 (Goldberg and Hillier 1979) but among patients with neurological disability a higher threshold of 12 or more is more valid (Bridges and Goldberg 1984, 1986).

Frequency of mood disturbance

Depressed mood after stroke seems common. Robinson and Price's early study (1982) found that 23 per cent of patients had GHQ scores of five or more, which they equated with a high prevalence of depression. However, the low threshold used tended to overestimate the true prevalence of depression. The study group was not typical of hospital or community practice. It included patients who were relatively young and the majority of whom were Black. Some had suffered strokes up to 10 years before, so it was possible that depression might well have resolved by this time, or be due to factors other than the initial stroke.

Recognizing the limitation of their first study the same authors collected 50 patients seen six months post-stroke and found that 60 per cent (95% CI 46–74%) (CI, confidence interval) were depressed (Robinson *et al.* 1984*a*). However, in this study they used different diagnostic criteria and unfortunately lost to follow-up over a third of the original consecutive series of patients. It was quite likely that selection bias occurred, leading to the more depressed patients returning for follow-up examinations, and thus a high depression prevalence.

Ebrahim *et al.* (1987*a*), using a threshold of 12 or more on the GHQ, reported a six-month mood disorder prevalence of 23 per cent (95% CI 16–30%) among a consecutive series of patients admitted to hospital with acute stroke. Follow-up losses were only 5 per cent, and only those with expressive dysphasia and cognitive impairment were excluded, and all were at home at the time of completing the GHQ. A much lower prevalence of psychiatric disorder (19 per cent with an abnormal score on the Present State

Examination—a structured psychiatric interview) was found in the Oxfordshire community study of stroke patients (House *et al.* 1989). By one year after the stroke this had fallen to 11 per cent. Diagnostic method and criteria, timing of measurements, together with selection bias can affect estimates of mood disorder markedly.

Depressed mood is quite common in people who have not had a stroke. In the United Kingdom, up to 36 per cent of women and 13 per cent of men aged 65–74 years report depressive symptoms (Ebrahim *et al.* 1988), so it is important to use a control group of unaffected subjects. In a study that has done this, depressive symptoms were about twice as common in stroke patients (six months after the event) compared with age and sex matched controls (Ebrahim *et al.* 1986).

Lesion location

Robinson and coworkers have claimed that the site of the stroke lesion is an important determinant of depressed mood; left hemisphere, more anterior lesions shown on CT scan were most strongly associated with depression (Robinson *et al.* 1984*b*). However, their correlation was very dependent on two subjects with very bad depression and anterior lesions, and the group included were only a small fraction of their total series. Attempts to replicate Robinson's work have failed (Sinyor *et al.* 1986; House pers. comm.), and no laterality effect was found in Ebrahim *et al.*'s study (1987*a*), suggesting that the observation may be a spurious result caused by selection bias.

Emotionalism

Emotional lability after stroke is common, but only one study has examined its frequency and causes (House *et al.* 1989). Lability, or 'emotionalism' affected one in five patients at six months and one in 10 patients at one year after their first stroke in the Oxfordshire Community Stroke Project. Although lability is thought to be common after bilateral strokes, it is clearly common after a single stroke. Lability was also strongly associated with the size of lesion on CT scanning, and with high mood scores, suggesting an association with depressed mood.

Causes of depression

Depression in old age is strongly associated with losses and life events (Murphy 1982) and post-stroke depression may well be a reaction to the loss of physical health and function. A small study comparing 20 stroke patients and 10 orthopaedic patients with similar levels of disability found that depression was more than four times as common in those with stroke (Folstein *et al.* 1977). A better comparison might have been with patients suffering a disease with an acute onset and an unpredictable prognosis. Mood disorder was strongly associated with both the extent of motor impairment and functional disability, and was worst in those whose disability increased over the first six months (Ebrahim *et al.* 1987*a*). This association with severity may explain why the Oxfordshire Community Stroke Study which included a higher proportion of less severe strokes found a lower prevalence of psychiatric disorder. However, many patients with minimal residual disability complained of depressed mood in both studies. Nabarro (1984) has drawn attention to this hidden problem of depression in medical patients arguing for increased psychiatric referral. A better policy would be the routine use of a depression questionnaire, such as the GHQ, and referral of those with high scores.

Treatment

At present, the majority of patients with depressed mood do not receive antidepressants when discharged from hospital (Ebrahim *et al.* 1987*a*), but are anti-depressants of any use? Only two trials of anti-depressant therapy after stroke have been published. The first, from Johns Hopkins University (Lipsey *et al.* 1984), used a double-blind, randomized design but suffered from a 33 per cent withdrawal rate among the 39 patients. This was compounded by an analysis of those remaining on treatment, rather than an intention to treat analysis (Schwartz and Lellouch 1967; Hampton 1981). The study was small with only 17 given the tricyclic anti-depressant, nortriptyline, and 22 on placebo. It included relatively young patients, and was concluded after only six weeks. Mood rating but not functional ability showed a fall in both groups, but a much bigger fall in those on active treatment. This was interpreted as a benefit from treatment but it is quite likely because of losses to follow-up and treatment withdrawals that those with only mild to moderate depression at the start of the study were the only ones still remaining on treatment at the end of the study. One correspondent pointed out that the only thing shown with any certainty in Lipsey's study was that nortriptyline is a toxic drug to give patients after a stroke (Agerholm 1984)!

A second treatment trial was reported by Redding and colleagues (1986) in which patients with and without depression (categorized in a variety of ways, including a dexamethasone suppression test) were randomized to either placebo (22 patients) or trazadone hydrochloride (25 patients). Treated patients were followed up for a week longer than placebo patients, with an overall trial length of about one month, thus treated patients had longer to improve. These investigators used the Barthel Activities of Daily Living scale as their outcome measure but were only able to show a significantly improved Barthel score in seven patients with an abnormal dexamethasone suppression test. The investigators stated that they studied a consecutive series of patients, yet the majority (89 per cent) had some evidence of depression. Although the anti-depressant used was meant to have fewer side-effects than older tricyclic compounds, a quarter of the patients were withdrawn because of side-effects. This study was unethical in concept because active, toxic treatment was given to patients who did not have any clinical indication for treatment. Sadly, the study does not contribute any useful information about the role of anti-depressant therapy after stroke.

The possible preventive effect of early and structured rehabilitation on post-stroke mood disorder has not been studied, and in view of the obvious toxicity of drug therapy in brain damaged people, it is surprising that none of the trials of stroke units versus usual care have used mood as an outcome measurement. It would be possible to set up a trial of the effect of extra emotional support and social engagement, perhaps included with drug therapy in a factorial design.

A small but properly designed trial of about 50 subjects in each group would be powerful enough to detect a treatment effect of about 50 per cent relative improvement in mood and ADL scores, assuming a similar measurement variance to that reported in these two studies. Much less toxic and probably lower doses of anti-depressant should be used in any further trials. Follow-up should be for much longer than a few weeks—most anti-depressants take at least two weeks to even begin to work. In the meantime, it is sensible to detect impaired mood using a questionnaire, refer patients with problems for psychiatric opinion, and if drug treatment is recommended, to use low doses of anti-depressants together with a supportive and encouraging rehabilitation programme.

Cognitive impairment

Adams and Hurwitz (1963) first drew attention to the poor rehabilitation prospects of patients suffering with cognitive impairment after a stroke. The size of this problem depends on the type of assessment of cognitive ability used. There is no general agreement about what abilities should be included under the heading of cognition. Most of the standard techniques used to assess 'cognition' focus mainly on short- and long-term memory, and orientation. All currently available assessment methods have been criticized because of failure to include items such as constructional apraxia, agnosia, verbal recall, nominal aphasia, auditory comprehension, and concept formation, and for their conceptual inadequacy (Ritchie 1988).

Most methods share common threads of short- and long-term memory and orientation in time, place and person. Short assessments agree with longer tests reasonably well (Hodkinson 1972) and are widely used. Despite its conceptual inadequacy (e.g. one of the items 'write a sentence' requires motor, psychomotor, visuospatial, visual scanning, and language skills), the Mini-Mental State examination (MMS) (Folstein *et al.* 1975) has some particular virtues: it covers a wider range of cognitive ability (orientation, registration, attention, calculation, recall, language, ability to follow a complex command, writing and copying a drawing) than the shorter tests; it is easy to use with stroke patients; patients may not find it as demeaning as the short tests (which include naming the Queen or Prime Minister and the year World War I began). However, it shares some of the problems of any pencil-and-paper test: it cannot be used with some dysphasic patients and it requires an attention span of at least 10 minutes.

The dilemma of where to draw the cut-off point between 'normal' and 'impaired' has been tackled, at least in part. The MMS was validated by comparisons with a physician's independent clinical assessments and with the Weschler Adult Intelligence Scale. The MMS is meant to 'separate patients with cognitive disturbance from those without such disturbance'. In fact, the MMS discriminates well between diagnostic *groups* but does not classify individuals so well.

Examination of the range of scores in each group gives an indication of the sensitivity and specificity of the MMS, the appropriate measurements for assessing the ability of a test to classify individuals. Normal subjects never scored below 24, and clear-cut demented subjects never scored above 21. A threshold of 24 or more would clearly separate out normal subjects. In practice, the clinical task is more subtle than this and tests are needed that will discriminate between dementia and depression. Depressed subjects scored anywhere from 8 to 30, the maximum. A threshold of 21 and below would pick up demented and depressed subjects with a sensitivity of 100 per cent; it would not permit discrimination between demented and depressed subjects. The MMS is of some use in describing the amount of cognitive impairment present but is not a diagnostic test. It must be supplemented with clinical observations and examination over a period of time.

In a consecutive series of 189 six month survivors of an acute stroke 12 per cent (95% CI 7–17%) of subjects had a MMS score below 22 out of 30, and in a third of these patients there was no prior evidence of dementia, cerebrovascular disease or depression (Ebrahim *et al.* 1985*a*). In subjects whose cognition declined between one and six months an association with depressed mood was found. Stroke severity was strongly associated with cognitive impairment which supports the view that the major determinant of cognitive impairment is the amount of brain damage (Tomlinson *et al.* 1970; Hachinski *et al.* 1985). A study among patients less than 65 years old reported a very similar level of 12 per cent suffering some impairment, with 6 per cent severe enough to satisfy DSM–III criteria for mild dementia (Kotila *et al.* 1986*a*).

Symptoms and signs of memory disturbance after stroke have been studied. Subjective complaint of memory impairment was more common amongst stroke patients than orthopaedic patients (Tinson and Lincoln 1987), and performance on story and picture memory was impaired in 29 per cent and 14 per cent respectively three months after a stroke (Wade *et al.* 1986*b*), although comparative data for these tests were not available. This leads to difficulty in deciding on a threshold for abnormality, consequently these prevalence estimates are arbitrary.

Fisher (1982) has reported six patients suffering a specific disorientation for place associated with right hemisphere parieto-occipital lesions, and in Ebrahim's study (1985) an excess of recall difficulty was found in patients with left hemisphere stroke. These observations suggest that the quality of cognitive impairment may well depend on the site of the brain damage.

Clinicians should assess cognition routinely, using the Mini-Mental State examination (Folstein *et al.* 1977) rather than the shorter, and less informative memory and orientation tests. They should consider the possibility of depressive illness in patients with impairments (Robinson *et al.* 1986). The effects of subjective memory impairment and learning difficulties on recovery require further study and the impact of memory retraining for those with less severe problems is not yet known but may hold some hope (Wilson 1982). The importance of advice and support for carers of cognitively impaired stroke patients and appropriate resettlement for badly affected patients should be obvious but, as with many aspects of stroke management, is often neglected (Ebrahim *et al.* 1987*b*).

Dysphasia

The frequency of dysphasia among early survivors varies from 10–16 per cent in community series (Hopkins 1975; Legh-Smith *et al.* 1987) to 33 per cent in hospital series (Marquardsen 1969). The prognosis for recovery among patients still dysphasic at 10 weeks is not good, with the majority of patients only making small improvements by six months (Lendrum and Lincoln 1985). Type of aphasia, age, and sex did not influence recovery.

Treatment

Three trials of speech therapy have been made, two making comparisons between professional and volunteer treatment (Meikle *et al.* 1979; David *et al.* 1982) and one with an untreated control group (Lincoln *et al.* 1984). The scale of improvement in all three trials was modest; scores on a Functional Communication Profile and the Porch Index of Communicative Ability rose by only a few points with no difference between speech therapy and volunteers or untreated controls. Drop-outs and those who recovered early were not included in the analyses which may tend to underestimate the true effects of therapy, but is unlikely to make a major change to the trial results. A curious finding in the Bristol trial (David *et al.* 1982) was that nine patients taken on long after the stroke (3 months to 2.5 years) showed exactly the same pattern of improvement as the rest. This has been interpreted as a genuine benefit of treatment as spontaneous recovery is very unlikely to occur by this time. However, it is quite possible that patients simply did better on the communication tests as they got used to them. The two baseline assessments for both early and late referrals showed an increasing trend prior to starting therapy which supports this interpretation.

As with any negative trial it is useful to examine the confidence intervals of the difference observed between comparison groups. The Bristol trial (David *et al.* 1982) compared 48 patients in each group and observed a difference of about 2 per cent in the Functional Communication Profile which has a standard deviation of about 20 per cent. The 95 per cent confidence intervals of this 2 per cent difference range from –6 per cent to 8 per cent. The Nottingham trial (Lincoln *et al.* 1984) had similar confidence intervals. Despite the relatively small size of these trials it is unlikely that an important treatment effect has been missed because such a precise measure of outcome was applied to every subject.

Speech therapists have responded, particularly to the Nottingham trial, claiming that the treatment given was too little, and started too late (after 10 weeks), that patients might have been unable to benefit because of deafness, dementia or other problems, and that the real questions are what methods and regimens of speech therapy are successful with which patients (Howard 1984; Williams *et al.* 1984). However, providing and attending intensive speech therapy is difficult; in Bristol only 5 per cent of those referred and 1 per cent of all cases of stroke were suitable for treatment five days a week (Legh-Smith *et al.* 1987). A case for the continued involvement of speech therapists with stroke patients has been made (Wade *et al.* 1985*a*) but with an emphasis on assessment, advising relatives, patients and staff, provision and instruction in use of communication aids, and organization of group activities for patients and relatives, although the cost-effectiveness of these recommendations has not been assessed.

Urinary incontinence

Incontinence after a stroke is a bad prognostic feature (Lorenze *et al.* 1959; Marquardsen 1969; Hurwitz and Adams 1972), but if patients survive their stroke, this condition tends to improve. The WHO stroke project (Aho *et al.* 1980) measured the occurrence of incontinence among a large but variably collected group of stroke patients. They found that 8 per cent were incontinent before the stroke, 25 per cent at three weeks, 14 per cent at three months, and only 10 per cent at one year. A New Zealand study of 151 hospital admitted patients also found a high prevalence of incontinence: 60 per cent at one week, 42 per cent at one month, and 29 per cent at three months after the stroke (Borrie *et al.* 1986). A similar pattern of falling prevalence after stroke was found by Brocklehurst and coworkers studying a selected group of patients (1985). In a community series (Wade and Hewer 1987) a lower prevalence was found; at three weeks and six months, 24 per cent and 11 per cent respectively were incontinent of urine, which is remarkably similar to the WHO series.

The prospect of recovering continence after stroke depends on the severity of the incontinence at one month. In Borrie *et al.*'s series (1986) two-thirds of those with only mild problems got better by three months, under a fifth of those with more severe incontinence had improved by this time, and an equal proportion had died. Incontinence before the stroke was not a bar to improvement in continence afterwards. The reduction in incontinence after a stroke is a result of spontaneous recovery among the mildly affected and death of the more severely incontinent.

Urinary incontinence is a common enough problem (Currie 1986), but what underlying mechanisms are responsible? Borrie *et al.*'s study (1986) used cystometry on those suffering with moderate or severe incontinence, and although only 19 patients were investigated it is the only study that has attempted this. Detrusor instability was the most frequent abnormality found but is common in old age and it may be a coincidental finding in stroke patients. As a control group was not studied concurrently it is difficult to comment on the importance of the cystometric results observed. It is quite possible that patients without incontinence have detrusor instability and that other factors (such as immobility, cognitive impairment, depression, site of lesion) must be present before incontinence results. Future studies should concentrate on examining urodynamics in both continent and incontinent patients, with consideration of these other important factors that may hinder achieving continence.

Treatment

Treatment of incontinence depends on its cause. Algorithms can be used to define various causes (Hilton and Stanton 1981) and the residual group may be assumed to have detrusor instability, although this may be unwarranted on present evidence. As the numbers of patients with persistent incontinence is relatively small, urodynamic studies should probably be carried out so that a precise diagnosis is reached. No specific treatment trials of incontinent stroke patients have been carried out so experience among other types of patients with detrusor instability must be used. Several studies have shown benefits from habit retraining (in which patients are taken to the toilet and encouraged to urinate every two hours, sometimes with the duration of time being extended as control improves), which may be augmented by use of anti-cholinergic drugs (Castleden *et al.* 1986).

A major problem with anti-cholinergics is their toxicity in brain damaged people. Newer, mixed calcium-channel blockers with mild anti-cholinergic activity may have a place (Tapp *et al.* 1987), but larger trials must be organized.

Single case study designs may well be helpful in assessing the use of various drugs for an individual patient if habit retraining is unsuccessful. A double blind design is feasible and incontinence may be recorded using a visual analogue scale or by nursing staff using the gradings of Castleden *et al.* (1986). The dangers of precipitating acute urinary retention and acute glaucoma are always present and patients should be carefully assessed before starting anti-cholinergic therapy.

Dysphagia

Choking on food and drink in the acute phase of both brainstem and hemisphere stroke is common. Up to 45 per cent of hospital admitted patients may have some evidence of dysphagia (Gordon *et al.* 1987) and among conscious patients about a third are affected initially (Barer 1984, 1987). Management of this serious complication varies from mandatory use of 'some alternative method of giving fluids' (Hewer 1987), 'swallowing therapy' (Barrett *et al.* 1987), to a 'wait and see' policy (Barer 1984). The presence and prognosis of dysphagia after hemisphere stroke probably depends on stroke severity, which should influence management. In the Bristol series (Gordon *et al.* 1987) 73 per cent of dysphagic patients also had some degree of impaired consciousness with an associated poor prognosis; overall, almost half the patients were dead within six weeks. Most survivors were able to swallow by two weeks. Maintaining hydration in drowsy, dysphagic patients may lead to survival of patients with a very poor prospect of improvement, and their high early death rate suggests that brain death rather than complications of dehydration is more important.

Barer's two hospital series are of interest as his patients had a relatively good prognosis (all unconscious patients were excluded) and were seen within 48 hours, the majority on the day of admission. One week after the stroke almost a half had recovered, a quarter had died and the rest were still affected to some degree (Barer 1984). In Barer's second series (1987) of 357 stroke patients, an analysis of the mortality of dysphagic patients, allowing for level of consciousness, showed that even alert dysphagic patients had an increased chance of dying (33 per cent dead by six months) compared with other alert stroke patients (7 per cent dead by six months).

It is not clear whether dysphagia during the acute phase causes significant dehydration leading to complications among survivors. Barer (1987) reported that changes in haematocrit and blood urea from admission to one week after the stroke were independent of dysphagia (and patients were not treated with intravenous fluids or naso-gastric tubes). Gordon and colleagues (1987) found that chest infections in the first week were more common among dysphagic patients (an 11 per cent difference, 95% CI 3–25%) but did not allow for impaired consciousness which might make infection more common. They asserted that naso-gastric tubes or intravenous fluids would prevent dehydration and chest infections, although there is no evidence to support the claim. It is quite possible that both of these practices could prove harmful, or lead to a reduced mortality but increased disability. In Barer's study (1987) pneumonia as a cause of death was equally common amongst those with and without dysphagia and dysphagic patients were twice as likely to suffer a primary brain death which probably reflects a simple association with stroke severity. Furthermore, the Scandinavian trial of haemodilution (Scandinavian Stroke Study Group 1987) did not produce any benefits and did not reduce the incidence of chest infections. It may be that maintaining hydration in badly affected patients does not affect the outcome.

A further analysis of dysphagic patients include in a trial of beta-blockade in acute stroke demonstrated that dysphagia was associated with a poor functional outcome at six months, even when several other severity variables were taken into account (Barer 1989). This suggests that dysphagia may have some influence on recovery that is independent of the initial severity of the stroke.

Treatment

Tube feeding is often tried for patients with persistent dysphagia. Selley (1985) makes a strong case against the use of naso-gastric tubes for stroke patients: (1) patients have to swallow, aspirate or drool about a litre of saliva a day and a naso-gastric tube is an effective method of increasing salivation; (2) a naso-gastric tube causes pharyngeal irritation which produces a peristaltic wave in the wrong direction hence counteracting the feedback needed for involuntary swallowing; (3) the tube can cause vomiting and aspiration; and (4) patients do not like naso-gastric tubes.

Selley has tested a new treatment for dysphagia. The 'palatal trainer' consists of a wire U-shaped loop fitted to the back of the patient's upper dental plate (or a small dental plate can be made if the patient has teeth), which rests along the soft palate and goes back almost to the uvula. It takes less than an hour to fit. Selley has tested this novel invention on a series of 170 consecutive stroke patients referred to him with dysphagia and drooling. Only 11 patients were referred acutely and the rest were seen months and even years after the stroke. In only six cases did the plate fail to stop drooling or choking. A randomized controlled trial would have given a much clearer answer about the true scale of benefit since most uncontrolled case series tend to overemphasize treatment effects. However, for most of these patients it is very unlikely that spontaneous recovery would have occurred simultaneously with insertion of the device at this late stage after the stroke. Moreover, some patients who removed the device early had a return of their symptoms, which was promptly resolved on replacing the device.

Management of dysphagia in the first two weeks is likely to remain controversial with the nihilists using a 'wait and see' approach and interventionists giving fluids. There is insufficient information to make a sound judgement on the issue. Naso-gastric tubes have many theoretical problems, therefore intravenous or subcutaneous hydration may be preferable in the small group of alert patients who have a relatively good prognosis, but suffer with persistent difficulty in swallowing. Selley's palatal training appliance should be tried in the management of dysphagia persisting longer than two weeks after stroke. Unconscious patients will continue to present a dilemma, although it is likely that maintaining hydration does not influence their outcome.

Some patients may suffer with persistent swallowing difficulty and be considered for long-term naso-gastric feeding or gastrostomy. One study has examined the indications and outcomes of such management (Ciocon *et al.* 1988). This study demonstrated a very high complication rate in patients with either type of tube. The major complications were aspiration pneumonia, need for restraint to keep the tube in place, and peritonitis in a few patients with gastrostomies. Tube-feeding did not prevent weight loss and was associated with a high mortality.

Deep vein thrombosis and pulmonary embolus

Several series of stroke patients have been investigated for deep vein thrombosis (Warlow *et al.* 1972; Denham *et al.* 1973; McCarthy *et al.* 1977). The common conclusion from these studies is that deep vein thrombosis (DVT) is very common, with an incidence of DVT in the first two weeks after a stroke of up to 75 per cent. Clinical diagnosis alone is not very sensitive, about 60 per cent in Warlow's series of 30 patients (1972), and although false-positive diagnoses are not likely to be common, the chances of correctly diagnosing DVT are around 50 per cent (Whitehouse 1987). This predictive value can be improved by a further clinical examination performed by a radiologist (Charig and Fletcher 1987).

Detecting clinically silent DVT can be difficult but investigation by new non-invasive tests such as liquid crystal thermography or ultrasound (Whitehouse 1987), which have much higher sensitivity than clinical examination and hence a greater negative predictive value, will increase the overall accuracy of diagnosis from around 60 to 98 per cent, which is a major advance. The consequences of recognizing this extra pathology are increased numbers of patients requiring anti-coagulation, the risks of bleeding, and the need for neuro-radiology to exclude haemorrhage as the cause of stroke prior to starting therapy.

Preventing DVT

Prevention is a much better option than diagnosing and treating established DVT. Prevention of DVT and pulmonary emboli by use of prophylactic low-dose heparin is effective after surgery (International Multicentre Trial 1975). This led McCarthy and Turner (1986) to investigate whether prophylaxis was effective after a stroke. As the risk of DVT is highest in the first week after a stroke treatment must begin early to stand any chance of success. They randomized any patient (without hypertension or contraindication to anti-coagulation) seen within 48 hours of a stroke to subcutaneous calcium heparin given 8 hourly for 14 days, but did not do CT scans to exclude patients with haemorrhages or haemorrhagic infarcts. Subcutaneous calcium heparin reduced the incidence of DVT from 73 per cent among controls to 22 per cent, and the 95 per cent confidence intervals of this difference of 51 per cent were 41–61 per cent. Pulmonary emboli diagnosed at post-mortem were reduced from 70 per cent among controls to 29 per cent. The overall 12 week mortality was also reduced from 33 to 22 per cent with this benefit limited to patients with less severe strokes. There was no excess risk of haemorrhage in those given heparin. Although the study was too small to detect even a large difference in haemorrhagic complications these are likely to be very small balanced against the benefits of treatment.

This study should be replicated in a larger series of patients to provide better estimates of the true risks of the treatment, with a longer observation period of six or more months. Patients who stay at home are unlikely to be offered this treatment because of the need for an 8 hourly regimen which would be beyond the resources of most community nursing services. Twice daily treatment with calcium heparin would be more practicable and acceptable both to staff and patients and is equally effective in other elderly patients (Walker *et al.* 1987), so should be used in future trials.

Quality of life

One of the major aims of rehabilitation is to increase a patient's quality of life, which may be equated with reducing handicap. Surprisingly, indicators of quality of life have not been used as outcomes of the effectiveness of specific interventions and yet may be more relevant than improvement in impairments, of physical disability and mortality (Seale and Davies 1987). A major problem has been the development of suitable measurement techniques (Walker and Rosser 1988).

Recent descriptive studies have assessed the impact of stroke on quality of life using a social activities index (the Frenchay Activities Index) for stroke patients (Wade *et al.* 1985*b*) and the Nottingham Health Profile (Ebrahim *et al.* 1986), which is a more general measurement of several dimensions (energy, pain, emotion, sleep, isolation, and mobility; together with effects of illness on normal life) of self-perceived health (Hunt *et al.* 1986). Such studies should be of use in highlighting problems that may be improved by rehabilitation, social or medical management.

The Frenchay Activities Index (FAI) consists of 15 activities, half of which are 'higher-order' activities of daily living (housework, walking, shopping), but also includes going out, gardening, reading, and work. The activities were chosen by a social worker rather than by enquiry from stroke patients or other people of activities done normally. Although the authors consider that the FAI is a 'valid, sensitive, reliable, communicable and relevant' measure, this conclusion stands on shaky ground. Comparisons were not made with other quality of life indicators, or with an age–sex matched control group. Reliability was only assessed in 14 patients and an overall correlation coefficient of 0.8 was used as an index of agreement, which is fallacious (Bland and Altman 1986), tending to hide the real extent of disagreement. Despite needing to modify criteria for doing an activity, further repeatability studies were not done. No data were presented on changes over time in individual patients, so the sensitivity to change of the FAI is not known. The FAI did highlight a possible reduction in driving and using public transport and an increase in social outings after the stroke. It is difficult to disentangle whether these findings are due to selection bias, advice and encouragement, or are part of the natural history of social recovery. The FAI requires considerable development work before it can be widely recommended.

By contrast the Nottingham Health Profile (NHP) was developed from statements made by people about the effects of illness on their quality of life. It has been extensively validated, tested for reliability, and sensitivity to intervention, and natural history of disease (Hunt *et al.* 1986). The NHP has been used with stroke patients admitted initially to hospital (Ebrahim *et al.* 1986). It is easy to use, and measured dimensions of illness experience that were independent of more objective indicators of disability, such as motor impairment and activities of daily living. Stroke patients more often lacked energy, felt depressed, were isolated and in pain than an age and sex matched control group. These problems were present one month after the stroke and tended to be worse by six months, even though most of the patients were at home by then.

It might be expected that patients with problems leading to a poor quality of life would receive more rehabilitation, medical and social attention. Unfortunately, this is not always the case. Hospital services (outpatient rehabilitation and medical clinics) were less often arranged for those with the worst NHP scores but domestic social support and home nursing were more closely related to apparent need (Ebrahim *et al.* 1986).

Although studies of the effectiveness of health and social services in improving quality of life have not yet been made, the descriptive studies reported do highlight how common problems are, show how such outcome measurements can be made, and also show that much more attention must be given to the targeting of services to those in most need. Problems such as pain and disturbed sleep need much more detailed systematic study to determine their causes and effective treatment.

Routine use of quality of life and disability measurements will undoubtedly increase awareness of the extent of a patient's difficulties. Until there are guidelines from trials of specific rehabilitation techniques individual goals should be set and progress monitored (using quality of life indicators as well as activities of daily living), and treatment (which may require several different skills) continued until goals are achieved or a plateau is reached.

Many patients' problems will not be solved by health and social services alone. An early study in Glasgow of the social consequences of stroke found that after discharge from hospital no patients went to the hairdresser, a library, or to places of entertainment (Isaacs *et al.* 1976). Innovative services must be developed aimed at improving various aspects of quality of life since these studies show that present rehabilitation falls far short of the desired goal of reducing handicap.

Carers of stroke patients

The life of many stroke patients is dependent on the person they live with, in most cases a spouse (Wade *et al.* 1986*a*; Ebrahim and Nouri 1987). The questions of how much support and for how long can carers be expected to give support, and how best can carers themselves be helped need to be answered. A small, very selected group of 13 spouses and patients living at home and interviewed at six months was reported by Field and colleagues (1983). The patients were not very disabled and this selection bias probably led to the conclusion that carers were 'coping with the practical problems . . . but all reported problems with emotional aspects of caring'. Study of a larger, consecutive series of patients living with someone would be a much more appropriate method to describe the extent of the burden of caring and the effects on the carer.

Even large studies of consecutive patients may run into problems if they ignore other sources of bias and do not make appropriate comparisons. A study reported from Bristol (Wade *et al.* 1986*a*) found that 11–13 per cent of carers were depressed (using the General Health Questionnaire) between six months and two years after the stroke. However, a higher threshold than that recommended (Goldberg and Hillier 1979) was used, which tended to underestimate the frequency of mood disorder. No comparison was made with an age and sex matched control group which was unfortunate because when used in general population surveys the General Health Questionnaire gives a high prevalence of mood disorder, around 27 per cent for people aged 18 to 64 (Freeling *et al.* 1985). Even clinical assessments by doctors yield high percentages (around 14 per cent) with psychiatric problems (Wilkinson *et al.* 1985). It might be concluded that carers of stroke patients had less mood disorder than expected!

The Bristol study may well have estimated unreliably the extent of carers' mood problems because of response bias. Although no response rates are reported, of 302 carers that could have been interviewed at one year after the stroke, 74 per cent were seen at six months, 78 per cent at one year, and 44 per cent at two years. Response bias may lead to those with fewest problems not being available for interview (perhaps because they were out working at the time), thus inflating the proportion with difficulties. A further source of bias in this study is due to selective survival of patients with less severe disability. This probably led to the authors finding no association between the patient's disability and the carer's mood at two years. Bereaved carers were not contacted which was a missed opportunity. The emotional needs of bereaved people may be met through counselling, but whether any impact can be made on their increased mortality (McAvoy 1986) is not known.

A smaller study done in Nottingham (Ebrahim and Nouri 1987) suffered less from selection and response bias. However, the patients studied had all been admitted to hospital initially and carers were only seen once six months later. A response rate of 98 per cent was achieved. Over two-thirds of carers had to give more care than before the stroke. Perhaps not surprisingly wives did more caring for more dependent spouses than husbands. Only a third of patients had been left unattended for all or part of the day prior to interview and almost one in five required help every night. Two-thirds of carers felt that this burden had had an adverse effect on their lives.

The limited role of health and social services in supporting carers has been demonstrated among elderly people in Wales (Jones and Vetter 1985), and this appears to be the case for stroke patients. Relief care (admission to an institution for a break, together with opportunity for rehabilitation, medical, and social therapy) tends to be offered to carers of less rather than more disabled people, and in the Nottingham series of patients, none had had a relief admission. Despite many patients being in touch with a 'service', patients and carers with bad problems were not picked up and referred. Hospital departments discharging patients should adopt some sort of follow-up and the family doctor must take a much more active role in the assessment and referral of those patients kept at home.

Summary

1. Mood disorder, usually depression, affects about a quarter of six month survivors. It frequently goes unrecognized but treatment with tricyclic anti-depressants is hazardous and of doubtful value. Alternatives to drug therapy should be sought.

2. Cognitive impairment affects about 12 per cent of six month survivors but underlying depressive illness may be responsible

rather than dementia. Specific treatment for milder memory and learning problems must be evaluated.

3. Dysphasia affects between 10 and 16 per cent of early survivors. Individual speech therapy does not lead to greater improvements than can be expected from spontaneous recovery alone.

4. Urinary incontinence is common early on (24 per cent affected at three weeks), but gets less common (11 per cent at six months) because of the combined effects of increased mortality and spontaneous improvement. The effectiveness of habit retraining, anticholinergic and calcium-channel blocking drugs have not been tested in stroke patients.

5. Dysphagia affects 45 per cent of acute stroke patients initially, falling to about 1 in 10 affected by two weeks. A palatal retraining wire should be tried for patients with persistent dysphagia. The value of naso-gastric tubes, parenteral hydration, and prophylactic antibiotics in reducing mortality and complications is not known.

6. Deep vein thrombosis affects up to three-quarters of hospital stroke patients, usually within the first two weeks of onset. Prevention with subcutaneous calcium heparin is feasible but requires further larger and longer trials to assess the risks of such therapy.

7. Quality of life is poor in many patients despite good physical recovery. More innovative programmes of social and psychological rehabilitation are needed.

8. Informal carers provide most of the support for patients and many do not get appropriate support despite being in touch with various health and social services. More systematic methods of routine follow-up are needed, together with improvements in the type and amount of support provided.

12 Recovery

Giving a prognosis for recovery is of obvious importance to patients and relatives. Prognostic information is also needed for deciding who should continue to have rehabilitation and should help in planning services and policy. Highlighting the problems of patients who make a poor recovery should make us look for new solutions and treatments. Indicators of recovery may also be used as a yardstick to audit the work done during rehabilitation.

Measuring recovery

The first question is: 'what is meant by recovery?' A conceptual framework for considering the impact of chronic disease has been produced by Wood and Badley (1978), and has resulted in the production of a WHO publication, the International Classification of Impairments, Disabilities and Handicaps (WHO 1980). Impairment is the physical or psychological lesion (e.g. hemianopia, hemiplegia); disability is the functional consequence of an impairment (e.g. inability to walk or dress); handicap is the consequence of disability given an individual's and the community's social, psychological, and health resources (e.g. social isolation because of inability to get outdoors). The concepts of impairment, disability and handicap are discussed more fully in Chapter 5 on severity. This model emphasizes the heterogeneous impact of chronic diseases, with an almost limitless combination of impairments, disabilities, and handicaps. However, many diverse impairments in stroke may lead to equally diverse types and degrees of handicap, but the number of possible disabilities is relatively small especially if ability for self-care is considered. Measurement of disability can therefore be applied to individuals with heterogeneous impairments and handicaps to produce relatively homogeneous groups of people with a much more limited range of disabilities. Estimates of recovery have to be made from pooling the experience of groups of patients, so the most commonly used indicator of recovery after stroke is achieving independence in self-care.

Activities of daily living

Disability has been assessed in different ways: motor ability; dependency on others; capacity for work and an ability for self and household care have all been used (Sainsbury 1973). Most methods of disability measurement deal only with self-care and go under the name of activities of daily living (ADL) scales. Most of the scales currently in use contain similar items (see Table 12.1) and there have been attempts to unify them (Donaldson *et al.* 1973; Jay 1976; Goble 1976). This has been unsuccessful because scales are used for different purposes. Assessments primarily for individual patients may be very detailed and time consuming whereas if the purpose of measurement is to examine the outcome of a group of patients then a short assessment containing key variables will be of more use. For example, it has been shown that walking, making tea, bathing, dressing, and transfer from floor to chair are the activities that explain most of the observed variation in the Northwick Park ADL Score (Sheikh *et al.* 1979).

Despite differences in items and scoring, comparisons between different ADL scales have shown high levels of agreement (Kelman and Willner 1962; Bebbington 1977) and appeared to classify very similar proportions of stroke patients as independent (Gresham *et al.* 1980).

A case has been made for stroke researchers to use the same indicator of disability so that comparisons between different research studies may be made more easily. The favoured indicator of some investigators is the Barthel scale (Wade 1986; Wade and Hewer 1987). The Barthel scale shares the same problems of most ADL scales: the maximum and minimum scores do not represent a patient's best and worst functional condition. Sensitivity to change, particularly at the less disabled end of the scale is small, which may lead to problems in detecting any benefits from rehabilitation among relatively fit patients. A further problem is that it is impossible to work out what a patient with a particular Barthel score can and cannot do, unless they score the minimum or maximum.

A ranked or hierarchical scale has the advantage that a scale score indicates which abilities a patient can and cannot do. It also has the advantage that not every item in an ADL assessment has to be tested. If patients cannot do items in the middle of a ranked scale it is highly unlikely that they will be able to do more difficult

Table 12.1 Comparison of items included in various ADL scales (+ = included)

Item	*Barthel*	*Northwick Park*	*Katz*	*Kenny*	*Rivermead*
Feeding	+	+	+	+	−
Drinking	−	−	−	−	+
Eating	−	−	−	−	−
Grooming	+	−	−	−	−
Clean teeth	−	+	−	−	+
Comb hair	−	+	−	−	+
Make up/shave	−	+	−	−	+
Wash face/hands	−	+	−	−	+
Dressing	+	+	+	+	−
Undress	−	−	−	−	+
Dress	−	−	−	−	+
Transfers					
Lie/sit	+	−	−	−	−
Bed/chair	+	+	+	+	+
Floor/chair	−	+	−	−	+
Mobility					
Indoor	+	+	+	+	+
Outdoor	−	+	−	−	+
Stairs	+	+	−	−	−
Use of toilet	+	+	+	+	+
Bathing					
Wash in bath	+	+	+	+	+
In/out bath	−	−	−	−	+
Overall wash	−	−	−	−	+
Using taps	−	+	−	−	−
Tea-making	−	−	−	−	+
Prepare for	−	+	−	−	−
Making tea	−	+	−	−	−
Continence	−	+	+	−	−
Bladder control	+	−	−	−	−
Bowel control	+	−	−	−	−

activities. Other benefits of ranking are that more information about types of disability is provided, people with the same scores can do the same activities and it is quicker to administer than a conventional additive scale as not all the items need to be tested. A ranked ADL scale has been developed for stroke patients (Whiting and Lincoln 1980; Ebrahim *et al.* 1985) and the Barthel scale using a different method of scoring from the original has hierarchical properties (Wade and Hewer 1987; see Chapter 5 on severity).

The Rankin grades of disability (Rankin 1957) have been widely used to report functional recovery, particularly among hospital series of patients (Marquardsen 1969; Adams and Hurwitz 1963; Adams 1975), and are shown in Table 12.2.

The major problems with Rankin grades are that the groupings—although rather crude—require some subjective judgement when allocating the patient to a grade and because the grades are broad it is not a very sensitive indicator of recovery. Moreover, patients may be unable to walk without help but able to 'attend to bodily needs', so the categories are not that easy to apply in practice.

As rehabilitation is concerned with reducing the degree of handicap patients experience, it has been argued that stroke rehabilitation involves several different outcomes: physical; functional; social; and emotional dimensions (Seale and Davies 1987). This will give a more complete picture of the effects of rehabilitation but may lead to the question of which outcome is of most importance. For

Table 12.2 Rankin grades of disability following stroke

Grade	*Functional ability*
I	No significant disability: able to carry out all usual duties
II	Slight disability: unable to carry out some of usual activities, but able to look after own affairs without assistance
III	Moderate disability: requires some help but able to walk without assistance
IV	Moderately severe disability: unable to walk without assistance, and unable to attend to own bodily needs without assistance
V	Severe disability: bed-ridden, incontinent, and requiring constant nursing care and attention

example, quality of life indicators are not coupled with improved physical ability (Ebrahim *et al.* 1986). For the purpose of reporting outcome after a stroke, many studies have simply compared the proportions independent with those dependent for various self-care activities (e.g. Garraway *et al.* 1980*a*, *b*). This makes comparisons difficult because different self-care activities may be used. It may lead to an inadequate appraisal of the true effects of rehabilitation as the severity of a stroke is the major determinant of subsequent physical ability rather than efforts at rehabilitation. In future clinical trials of rehabilitation and natural history studies should aim to measure several dimensions of outcome.

A further problem is that in several widely quoted sources the time at which observations were made is not stated (Rankin 1957; Marquardsen 1969; Adams and Hurwitz 1963). As recovery is a time-dependent function, it is essential that observations be made at points after onset if the observations are to be of any use. The question of whether to include or exclude patients who die from the denominator when calculating percentage of recovery also arises. An apparent increase in independence may be achieved by the more disabled patients dying, rather than disabled people getting better. It is essential, therefore, when examining the rate of recovery either to consider only patients who survived for the whole time interval, thus ensuring that the denominator stays the same, or alternatively, the proportion dying during each time interval should be stated. The use of life table methods is most appropriate with the time taken to reach a rehabilitation 'milestone'. This permits adjustment of the denominator by taking account of deaths along the way, thus giving a valid assessment of the true rate of recovery. This approach could be developed to produce charts with a median recovery rate together with boundaries for 90th and 10th centiles, in a similar manner to child health growth charts. Patients not progressing at an average or better rate might then be singled out for careful assessment.

Pattern of recovery

The proportion of patients achieving independence in self-care by one year after a stroke ranges from 60 per cent (Aho *et al.* 1980) to 69 per cent (Andrews *et al.* 1981) in community series; from 38 per cent (Stevens *et al.* 1984) to 68 per cent (Kotila *et al.* 1984) in hospital series; and from 60 per cent (Bernspang 1987) to 83 per cent (Skilbeck *et al.* 1983) among rehabilitation patients. Data from these and other studies are shown in Table 12.3.

Why should estimates be so variable? The precision of the estimates shown in Table 12.3 demonstrates that chance alone is not the sole explanation. The community series are less variable probably because of less selection bias in the severity of cases considered. The proportion classified as independent will also depend on the activities considered. For example, in Wade and Hewer's study (1987), 85 per cent were independent in walking but only 47 per cent were independent in all activities of daily living. Stevens *et al.* (1984) used only four activities (washing, toileting, dressing, and eating), and yet found one of the lowest levels of independence of any published series. Most studies give very little detail about how ability was measured yet the method used to rate ability will affect the level of dependency found. Nurses tend to rate patients as more disabled than formal assessments done by an occupational therapist (Ebrahim *et al.* 1985*b*).

There is much greater agreement in the place of residence after a stroke, which reflects dependency to some extent (see Table 12.4). Presumably this is because differences in criteria and method do not have an effect. Surprisingly good agreement between community and hospital series is found, with about one in five survivors resident in an institution at one year.

The rate of recovery has been measured in small series of patients seen regularly (Skilbeck *et al.* 1983; Andrews *et al.* 1981; Partridge *et al.* 1987). The bulk of spontaneous recovery occurs in the first three months after the stroke, with some continued improvement up to six months and little change after this. This appears to be so for both overall ability in self-care and also for language recovery and motor recovery (Skilbeck *et al.* 1983). Although it is well recognized that some patients can continue to improve for up to two years, large systematic studies of long-term recovery have not been done.

The recovery of very severely affected stroke patients is of great importance because these groups often receive a lot of rehabilitation effort without much apparent benefit (Brocklehurst *et al.* 1978; Andrews *et al.* 1982*a*). Even in such patients over half may make some improvement over the first year. The bulk of this improvement occurs in the first six months, with only 6 per cent of survivors

Table 12.3 The percentage of survivors of stroke achieving independence in self-care and other specified activities at various times after the stroke

Study	*Time since stroke*	*Percentage independent (95% CI)*
Community patients		
Aho *et al.* (1980)	3 mths	51 (50–52)
	1 yr	60 (59–61)
Andrews *et al.* (1981)	6 mths	70 (61–79)
	1 yr	69 (59–79)
Gresham *et al.* (1979)	6 mths–4 yrs	68 (60–76)
Wade and Hewer (1987)	6 mths	47 (43–51)
	in a transfer	81 (78–84)
Weddell and Beresford (1979)	3 mths	
	in a transfer	71 (63–79)
Hospital patients		
Allen (1984*b*)	2 mths	56 (48–64)
	6 mths	66 (58–74)
Garraway *et al.* (1980*b*)	1 yr	57 (47–67)
Henley *et al.* (1985)	1 yr	55 (45–65)
Kotila *et al.* (1984*a*)	3 mths	62 (54–70)
	1 yr	68 (61–75)
Stevens *et al.* (1984)	1 yr	38 (29–47)
	in walking	67 (58–76)
Rehabilitation patients		
Bernspang (1987)	4–6 yrs	60 (48–71)
Kinsella and Ford (1985)	4 wks	32 (16–48)
	8 wks	58 (41–75)
	12 wks	71 (55–87)
	1+ yrs	75 (60–90)
Skilbeck *et al.* (1983)	3 mths	71 (62–80)
	6 mths	81 (73–89)
	1 yr	83 (75–91)

Table 12.4 Percentage of survivors of stroke resident in an institution at various times after the stroke

Study	*Time*	*Percentage resident in an institution (95% CI)*
Community patients		
Aho *et al.* (1980)	3 wks	65 (63–67)
	3 mths	25 (24–26)
	1 yr	16 (15–17)
Gresham *et al.* (1975, 1979)	6 mths–4 yrs	15, 16 (10–21)
Weddell and Beresford (1979)	3 mths	30 (22–38)
Hospital patients		
Barer (1987)	1 mth	60 (56–64)
	6 mths	18 (13–23)
Kotila *et al.* (1984)	3 mths	31 (24–38)
	1 yr	22 (16–28)
Stevens *et al.* (1984)	1 yr	22 (14–30)
Rehabilitation patients		
Bernspang (1987)	4–6 yrs	14 (6–22)
Isaacs and Marks (1973)	1 yr	31 (23–39)

improving to the point of walking with aids by one year (Andrews *et al.* 1981). However, these figures hide the fact that if a patient is unable to walk at six months the chance of walking by one year is 40 per cent. Moreover, more modest improvements, such as requiring one helper instead of two have not been reported, and yet have a great impact on possibilities for resettlement. It would be unwise to ration rehabilitation resources after six months as suggested (Andrews *et al.* 1981) without more detailed studies.

Recovery of the ability to roll over in bed, sitting balance, transfer from bed to chair, and walking, among patients referred for rehabilitation appear to follow a very predictable pattern over the first eight weeks (Partridge *et al.* 1987). Therefore it may be possible to produce an expected profile against which individual patients' progress may be compared. This would be of use in identifying patients whose recovery was slower than expected, would allow goals to be set, and should lead to identification of factors limiting progress. Such an approach would be most useful in examining the question of continued rehabilitation for severely affected stroke patients.

The indicators of recovery used limit the detection of small but important improvements and also reach a ceiling which does not correspond to maximum ability. These problems could be overcome by using more sensitive grades of dependency and adding more complex activities to the top of the scale. A greater problem is the need to consider recovery of other dimensions of life, besides physical function. For example, at six months post-stroke Nottingham Health Profile scores are about two to four times higher than expected, indicating important problems (such as social isolation, lack of energy, emotional upset), and yet most patients are at home by this time, and most are independent in a majority of activities of daily living (Ebrahim *et al.* 1986).

Problems persist for a long time; survivors of stroke in the Framingham study showed decreased interest in hobbies and difficulty using transport up to four years after the stroke (Gresham *et al.* 1979). A study of patients discharged from a stroke rehabilitation unit found that almost two-thirds of patients had decreased life satisfaction (usually concerned with general, sexual, and leisure satisfaction) four to six years later (Bernspang 1987). As rehabilitation aims to improve specific impairments, functional abilities, and handicap it will be necessary in future to examine the natural history of recovery of not just physical disability but other aspects of quality of life.

Predictors of recovery

Ideally, predictors for types of stroke, different severities and for a range of indicators of recovery (recovery of impairments, disabilities, and handicap) are needed. In practice, there are reports on the predictors of recovery of only aphasia (Lendrum and Lincoln 1985) and arm function (Wade *et al.* 1983*b*; Heller *et al.* 1987). The natural history of hemi-inattention (Kinsella and Ford 1985), of visual neglect (Kotila *et al.* 1986*b*; Sunderland *et al.* 1987), of motor function (Skilbeck *et al.* 1983) has been described but prediction of recovery of these and other impairments has not been attempted.

Most work has been done on predicting death (see Chapter 9 on mortality) and physical ability using activities of daily living scales. Very little work has been done on predicting the quality of life of stroke patients (Ebrahim *et al.* 1986; Bernspang 1987). Numerous factors have been described which influence the functional outcome of stroke patients (see Table 12.5). These may be classified as those concerned with the site and extent of the lesion (Andrews *et al.* 1980; Andrews *et al.* 1982*b*), with complications of the stroke, and with other factors, such as mood and morale, pre-stroke morbidity, social factors, and age.

Guy's Hospital prognostic score

As many of these variables are interrelated, a search has been made for those factors that appear to independently predict outcome. The Guy's Hospital prognostic score (Allen 1984*b*) comprises degree

Table 12.5 Predictors of dependence in functional ability among survivors of an acute stroke

Site and extent of lesion	*Other factors*	*Complications*
Severe motor deficit	Age	Urinary incontinence
Sensory inattention	Sex	Pneumonia
Balance/posture	Marital status	Hypotension
ADL in first month	Previous stroke	
Proprioception	Pre-stroke immobility	
Impaired consciousness	Mood	
Duration of unconsciousness	Poor motivation	
Flaccidity		
Hemisensory loss		
Bilateral signs		
Visuo-spatial impairment		
Memory impairment		
Aphasia		
Right hemisphere lesion		
Gaze paresis		
Nystagmus		

of paralysis, 'complicated stroke' (i.e. higher cerebral dysfunction, hemianopia, and hemiplegia), loss of consciousness at onset, impaired consciousness for more than 24 hours, and age. It correctly classified 92 per cent of 'good' outcomes and 84 per cent of 'bad' outcomes at two months. However, this scoring system was developed in patients under 76 years old, did not examine the influence of predictors later in the course of recovery and included death as a bad outcome. This last point probably explains the importance of impaired consciousness in the score as 58 per cent of the 'bad' outcomes at two months were due to death. The 'good' outcomes were largely those patients able to walk. Social, emotional, and pre-stroke factors were not considered. The Guy's Hospital prognostic score needs to be tested on another series of patients (to replicate the scoring used), in a wider age range of patients, over a longer time period, and with functional ability and death examined separately before it can be recommended as a useful prognostic index.

The Bristol prognostic score

The Bristol prognostic score (Wade *et al.* 1983*a*) was derived from 83 patients referred for rehabilitation. It comprises age, presence of hemianopia or visual inattention, urinary incontinence, severity of motor deficit in the arm, and sitting balance. Of these measurements, 89 per cent were made within the first month, but only 20 per cent within the first week after onset. The score aimed to predict Barthel scores at six months, but only predicted 38 per cent of the variance and was accurate to +/− 5 Barthel points in 55 per cent of patients. Although the authors claimed that this was better than any other method, Britton *et al.* (1980) showed that the admitting doctor made a correct functional prognosis in 59 per cent of cases without the aid of any scoring system.

When the Bristol system was tested in another group of patients, with measurements made at a set time after stroke, and using data from a community series of patients (Wade and Hewer 1987) different factors were important: urinary incontinence; initial Barthel score; age; and sitting balance, measured within one week predicted 26 per cent of the variance in six month Barthel scores, but incorrectly classified at least a third of patients (correct classifications were included with under-predictions). At three weeks after the stroke IQ (measured using Raven's matrices) and Barthel score together with urinary incontinence, age, sitting balance, and arm motor function accounted for 29 per cent of the variance in six month Barthel scores but still incorrectly predicted scores in over a third of the patients. The analyses were restricted to patients with some disability at the time of being seen, so it is uncertain whether the index will predict deterioration in patients with minimal or no disability. Social and emotional factors, and pre-stroke disability should also be considered and since so little of the variance in Barthel scores was explained it is quite possible that other more important predictors of functional outcome exist.

Other predictors of recovery

Urinary incontinence, age, extensive motor deficit, and combined neurological deficits are important predictors of functional ability at discharge from hospital (Sheikh *et al.* 1983; Wade *et al.* 1984*c*; Wade *et al.* 1985*c*). Disability from a previous stroke, and female sex also had an adverse effect, but only accounted for 18 per cent of the variation in ability at discharge. Arm motor function, proprioception (thumb finding) and 'postural function' (i.e. sitting and standing balance, and walking) were the most important factors among a group of patients admitted to a stroke unit (Prescott *et al.* 1982). In this case, the outcome used was 'reaching independence' which could be achieved at any point in time up to 16 weeks. Patients with minor and devastating strokes had been excluded, so these predictors of recovery do not reflect the range of severity seen in patients admitted to hospital. Furthermore, the length of follow-up was too short and variable to be certain that these factors would have a lasting adverse influence.

Among a series of patients admitted to hospital and followed up for six months, urinary incontinence, sensory inattention, pre-stroke mobility, severity of motor deficit, and age, predicted 58 per cent of the variation in six month activities of daily living scores. Addition of one month ADL scores improved the prediction to 66 per cent and classified 69 per cent of patients to within 1 scale point of the activities of daily living score. Half of the variation in six month activities of daily living scores was explained by just three factors: persisting urinary incontinence; sensory inattention; and pre-stroke immobility (Ebrahim 1985). These factors are easy to measure and should be applicable to hospital admitted stroke patients (rather than those referred for rehabilitation, or community patients). Their predictive power has been replicated in another hospital series (Barer and Mitchell 1989).

Predictors need deeper understanding. For example, the reasons for urinary incontinence may include immobility, cognitive failure, loss of morale, too few toilets, constipation, and urinary infection, some of these could be responsible for a poor prognosis. Alternatively, incontinence may simply reflect stroke severity. Sensory inattention also requires further study. Small studies have shown that even amongst those who recover attention, their ADL recovery is worse than expected (Kinsella and Ford 1985; Kotila *et al.* 1986*b*), and the adverse effects of perceptual impairments is long lasting (Bernspang 1987).

The impact of other diseases (e.g. Parkinsonism, osteoarthritis, heart failure, etc.) causing poor mobility and function before the stroke must be reduced by diagnosis and treatment, but often such problems are overlooked in the face of the stroke. This should not come as any surprise to geriatricians but it is comforting that standard practice of making a complete assessment, setting priorities, and treating problems is actually reflected in a multivariate regression that demonstrates that pre-stroke problems have an impact on outcome.

Predicting independent life outside an institution is a less ambitious task than prediction of a range of activities of daily living, but nonetheless, is useful. The two studies that have tried to do this have included measures of disability in the prediction equations. Not surprisingly, independent life is more likely if the patient has a good level of functional ability (Dejong and Branch 1982; Henley *et al.* 1985). These studies highlighted an important contribution of mood and marital status in determining independence. It would also be of use to examine predictors of independent life among severely affected patients, and those referred for rehabilitation. Choice of which potential predictors to consider should be guided by considering whether they may be modifiable either by health service or social intervention, and the ease with which they can be measured.

Summary

1. The pattern of recovery after stroke is very variable, depending

on the patients considered, the criteria used to define independence, and the time at which observations are made. Best estimates for survivors from community series are 45 per cent independent at six months and about 60 per cent independent at one year. Hospital series range from 38 to 68 per cent independent at one year. Around 20 per cent of survivors are in an institution at one year after the stroke.

2. More standard methods of reporting disability, dependency, and the social and emotional consequences of stroke are needed. Without standard methods it is impossible to compare studies and our understanding of the pattern of recovery will remain limited to physical aspects of disability. This may lead to underestimation of the effects of treatment.

3. The bulk of recovery of physical ability in self-care appears to occur over the first six months and is most rapid over the first three months. However, among the very disabled, almost half show improvements between six months and one year. No studies have examined rate of recovery beyond this time but since these patients are often receiving rehabilitation this needs to be done. The rate of recovery of other aspects of life has not been studied.

4. The main predictors of recovery of physical ability for self-care at six months are: severity of the stroke; urinary incontinence; sensory inattention; pre-stroke mobility; balance; and arm motor deficit, measured in the first week. Predictors among severely affected patients and those referred for rehabilitation are needed. Predictors of other aspects of handicap (especially emotional and social outcomes) are needed.

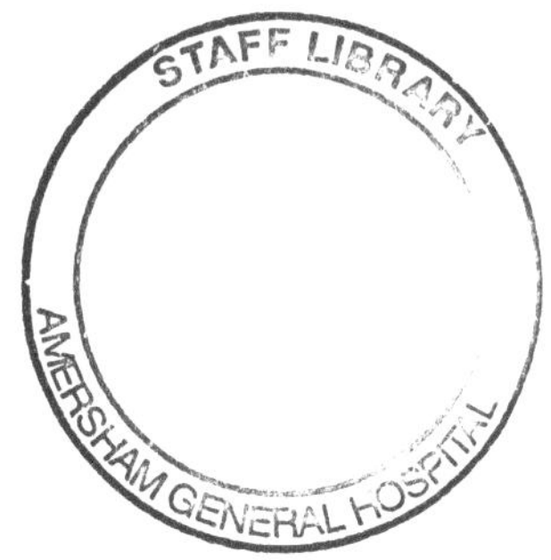

References

Acheson, R.M. and Sanderson, C. (1978). Strokes: social class and geography. *Population Trends*, **12**, 13–17.

Acheson, R.M. and Williams, D.D.R. (1980). Epidemiology of cerebrovascular disease: some unanswered questions. In *Clinical neuroepidemiology* (ed. F.C. Rose), pp. 88–104. Pitman Medical, London.

Acheson, R.M. and Williams, D.R.R. (1983). Does consumption of fruit and vegetables protect against stroke? *Lancet*, **1**, 1191–3.

Adams, G.F. (1965). Prospects for patients with strokes, with special reference to the hypertensive hemiplegic. *British Medical Journal*, **2**, 253–9.

Adams, G.F. (1975). Grading of functional recovery from strokes. *Age and Ageing*, **4**, 137–41.

Adams, G.F. and Merrett, J.D. (1961). Prognosis and survival in the aftermath of hemiplegia. *British Medical Journal*, **1**, 309–14.

Adams, G.F. and Hurwitz, L.J. (1963). Mental barriers to recovery from stroke. *Lancet*, **2**, 533–7.

Agerholm, M. (1984). Side-effects of nortriptyline treatment for post-stroke depression. *Lancet*, **1**, 519–20.

Aho, K., Harmsen, P., Hatano, S. *et al.* (1980). Cerebrovascular disease in the community: results of a WHO Collaborative Study. *Bulletin of the World Health Organization*, **58**, 113–30.

Alfredsson, L., von Arbin, M., and De Faire, U. (1986). Mortality from and incidence of stroke in Stockholm. *British Medical Journal*, **292**, 1299–1303.

Allen, C.M.C. (1983). Clinical diagnosis of the acute stroke syndrome. *Quarterly Journal of Medicine, NS*, **LII**, 515–23.

Allen, C.M.C. (1984*a*). Predicting recovery after acute stroke. *British Journal of Hospital Medicine*, **31**, 428–34.

Allen, C.M.C. (1984*b*). Predicting the outcome of acute stroke: a prognostic score. *Journal of Neurology, Neurosurgery and Psychiatry*, **47**, 475–80.

Allen, C.M.C. (1984*c*). Differential diagnosis of acute stroke: a review. *Journal of Royal Society of Medicine*, **77**, 878–81.

Amery, A., Birkenhager, W., Brixko, P. *et al.* (1985). Mortality and morbidity results from the European Working Party on High Blood Pressure in the Elderly trial. *Lancet*, **1**, 1349–54.

Amery, A., Birkenhager, W., Brixko, P. *et al.* (1986). Efficacy of anti-hypertensive drug treatment according to age, sex, blood pressure, and previous cardiovascular disease in patients over the age of 60. *Lancet*, **2**, 589–92.

Andrews, K., Brocklehurst, J.C., Richards, B., and Laycock, P.J. (1980). The prognostic value of picture drawings by stroke patients. *Rheumatology and Rehabilitation*, **19**, 180–8.

Andrews, K., Brocklehurst, J.C., Richards, B., and Laycock, P.J. (1981). The rate of recovery from stroke—and its measurement. *International Rehabilitation Medicine*, **3**, 155–61.

Andrews, K., Brocklehurst, J.C., Richards, B., and Laycock, P.J. (1982*a*). The recovery of the severely disabled stroke patient. *Rheumatology and Rehabilitation*, **21**, 225–30.

Andrews, K., Brocklehurst, J.C., Richards, B., and Laycock, P.J. (1982*b*). Stroke: does side matter. *Rheumatology and Rehabilitation*, **21**, 175–8.

Anonymous (1983). Why has stroke mortality declined? *Lancet*, **1**, 1195–6.

Anonymous (1985). Treatment of hypertension: the 1985 results. (Editorial) *Lancet*, **2**, 645–7.

Anonymous (1987*a*). Consensus on heart failure management. *Lancet*, **2**, 311–13.

Anonymous (1987*b*). Steroids in haemorrhagic stroke. *Lancet*, **2**, 547–8.

Antiplatelet Trialists' Collaboration (1988). Secondary prevention of vascular disease by prolonged antiplatelet treatment. *British Medical Journal*, **296**, 320–1.

Aring, G.C.D. and Merritt, M.H. (1935). Differential diagnosis between cerebral haemorrhage and thrombosis. *Archives of Internal Medicine*, **56**, 435–56.

Baker, R., Broward, J., Fang, H. *et al.* (1962). Anticoagulant therapy in cerebral infarction: report on cooperative study. *Neurology*, **12**, 823–9.

Bamford, J. and Warlow, C. (1988). Evolution and testing the lacunar hypothesis. *Stroke*, **19**, 1074–82.

Bamford, J., Sandercock, P., Warlow, C., and Gray, M. (1986). Why are patients with acute stroke admitted to hospital. *British Medical Journal*, **292**, 1369–72.

Bamford, J., Sandercock, P., Dennis, M. *et al.* (1988). A prospective study of acute cerebrovascular disease in the community: the Oxfordshire Stroke Project 1981–86. 1. Methodology, demography, and incident cases of first-ever stroke. *Journal of Neurology, Neurosurgery, and Psychiatry*, **51**, 1373–80.

Bamford, J., Sandercock, P., Warlow, C.P., and Slattery, J. (1989). Interobserver agreement for the assessment of handicap in stroke patients. *Stroke*, **20**, 828.

Barer, D.H., Ebrahim, S., and Smith, C. (1984). Factors affecting the day to day incidence of stroke in Nottingham. *British Medical Journal*, **289**, 662.

Barer, D.H. (1984). Lower cranial nerve function in unilateral vascular lesions of the cerebral hemisphere. *British Medical Journal*, **289**, 1622.

Barer, D.H. (1987). Dysphagia in acute stroke. *British Medical Journal*, **295**, 1137–8.

Barer, D.H. (1989). The natural history and functional consequences of dysphagia after hemispheric stroke. *Journal of Neurology, Neurosurgery, and Psychiatry*, **52**, 236–41.

Barer, D.H. and Mitchell, J.R.A. (1989). Predicting the outcome of acute stroke: do multivariate models help? *Quarterly Journal of Medicine*, *NS 70*, **261**, 27–39.

Barer, D.H., Ebrahim, S., and Mitchell, J.R.A. (1988*a*). The pragmatic approach to trial design: stroke register, pilot trial, assessment of neurological then functional outcome. *Neuroepidemiology*, **7**, 1–12.

Barer, D.H., Cruickshank, J.M., Ebrahim, S.B., and Mitchell, J.R.A. (1988*b*). Low dose beta-blockade in acute stroke ('BEST' trial): an evaluation. *British Medical Journal*, **296**, 737–41.

Barker, D.J.P. and Osmond, C. (1987). Death rates from stroke in England and Wales predicted from past maternal mortality. *British Medical Journal*, **295**, 83–6.

Barrett, J.A., Fullerton, K.J., Wyatt, R., and O'Neill, P.A. (1987). Dysphagia in acute stroke. *British Medical Journal*, **295**, 1137.

Baskin, D.S. and Hosobuchi, Y. (1981). Naloxone reversal of ischaemic neurological defecits in man. *Lancet*, **2**, 272–5.

Baum, M. (1987). Endoscopic coagulation of upper gastrointestinal haemorrhage, one; randomised clinical trials, two. *British Medical Journal*, **295**, 212.

Bayer, A.J., Pathy, M.S.J., and Newcombe, R. (1987). Double-blind randomised trial of intravenous glycerol in acute stroke. *Lancet*, **1**, 405–8.

Bebbington, A.C. (1977). Scaling indices of disablement. *British Journal of Preventive and Social Medicine*, **31**, 122–6.

Beevers, D., Fairman, M., Hamilton, M. *et al.* (1973). Antihypertensive treatment and the course of established cerebral vascular disease. *Lancet*, **1**, 1407–9.

Bernspang, B. (1987). Consequences of stroke. Aspects of impairments, disabilities, and life satisfaction. With special emphasis on perception and on occupational therapy. *Umea University Medical Disertations*, *NS 202*, Umea, Sweden.

Blackburn, H., Blomgvist, G., Freiman, A. *et al.* (1968). The exercise electrocardiogram: differences in interpretation. Report of a technical group on exercise electrocardiography. *American Journal of Cardiology*, **21**, 871–80.

Bland, J.M. and Altman, D.G. (1986). Statistical methods for assessing agreement between two methods of clinical measurement. *Lancet*, **1**, 307–10.

Bleuler, E.P. (1924). *Textbook of psychiatry*, p. 280. MacMillan, New York.

Bobarth, B. (1970). *Adult hemiplegia: evaluation and treatment.* William Heinemann, London.

Boers, G.H.J., Smals, A.G.H., Tribjbels, F.J.M. *et al.* (1985). Heterozygosity of homocystinuria in premature peripheral and cerebral occlusive arterial disease. *New England Journal of Medicine*, **313**, 709–15.

Bonita, R. and Beaglehole, R. (1986). Does treatment of hypertension explain the decline in mortality from stroke? *British Medical Journal*, **292**, 191–2.

Bonita, R., Beaglehole, R., and North, J.D.K. (1984). Event, incidence and case fatality rates of cerebrovascular disease in Auckland, New Zealand. *American Journal of Epidemiology*, **120**, 236–43.

Bonita, R., Scragg, R., Stewart, A., Jackson, R., and Beaglehole, R. (1986). Cigarette smoking and risk of premature stroke in men and women. *British Medical Journal*, **293**, 6–8.

Borrie, M.J., Campbell, A.J., Caradoc-Davies, T., and Spears, G.F.S. (1986). Urinary incontinence after stroke: a prospective study. *Age and Ageing*, **15**, 177–81.

Bousser, M.G., Eschwege, E., Haguenau, M. *et al.* (1983). AICLA controlled trial of aspirin and dipyridamole in the secondary prevention of atherothrombotic cerebral ischaemia. *Stroke*, **14**, 5–14.

Brennan, P.J., Greenberg, G., Miall, W.E., and Thompson, S.G. (1982). Seasonal variation in blood pressure. *British Medical Journal*, **285**, 919–23.

Bridges, K. and Goldberg, D. (1984). Psychiatric illness in inpatients with neurological disorders, patients' views on discussion of emotional problems with neurologists. *British Medical Journal*, **289**, 656–8.

Bridges, K. and Goldberg, D. (1986). The validation of the GHQ-28 and the use of the Mini-Mental State Examination in neurological inpatients. *British Journal of Psychiatry*, **148**, 548–53.

Britton, M., Faire, U. de, Helmers, C., and Miah, K. (1980*a*). Prognostication in acute cerebrovascular disease. *Acta Medica Scandinavica*, **207**, 37–42.

Britton, M., Faire, U. de, Miah, K., and Rane, A. (1980*b*). Lack of effect of theophylline on the outcome of acute cerebral infarction. *Acta Neurologica Scandinavica*, **62**, 116–23.

Britton, M., Hultman, E., Murray, V., and Sjoholm, H. (1983). The diagnostic accuracy of CSF analyses in stroke. *Acta Medica Scandinavica*, **214**, 3–13.

Brocklehurst, J.C., Andrews, K., Richards, B., and Laycock, P.J. (1978). How much physical therapy for patients with stroke. *British Medical Journal*, **1**, 1307–10.

Brocklehurst, J.C., Andrews, K., Richards, B., and Laycock, P.J. (1985). Incidence and correlates of incontinence in stroke patients. *Journal of the American Geriatrics Society*, **33**, 540–2.

Broderick, J.P., Phillips, S.J., Whisnant, J.P., O'Fallon, W.M., and Bergstralh, E.J. (1989). Incidence rates of stroke in the Eighties: the end of the decline in stroke? *Stroke*, **20**, 577–82.

Bucknall, C.A., Morris, G.K., and Mitchell, J.R.A. (1986). Physicians' attitudes to four common problems: hypertension, atrial fibrillation, transient ischaemic attacks, and angina pectoris. *British Medical Journal*, **293**, 739–42.

Canadian Cooperative Study Group (1978). A randomised trial of aspirin and sulfinpyrazone in threatened stroke. *New England Journal of Medicine*, **299**, 53–9.

Carter, A.B. (1961). Anticoagulant treatment in progressing stroke. *British Medical Journal*, **2**, 70–3.

Carter, A.B. (1964). *Cerebral infarction*. London, Pergamon Press.

Carter, A.B. (1970). Hypotensive therapy in stroke survivors. *Lancet*, **1**, 485–9.

Castleden, C.M., Duffin, H.M., and Gulati, R.S. (1986). Double blind study of imipramine and placebo for incontinence due to bladder instability. *Age and Ageing*, **15**, 299–303.

Cerebral Embolism Study Group (1983). Immediate anticoagulation of embolic stroke: a randomised trial. *Stroke*, **14**, 668–76.

Chalmers, T., Matta, R., Smith, H., and Kunzler, A. (1977). Evidence favouring the use of anticoagulants in the hospital phase of acute myocardial infarction. *New England Journal of Medicine*, **297**, 1091–6.

Charig, M.J. and Fletcher, E.W.L. (1987). Emergency phlebography service: is it worthwhile. *British Medical Journal*, **295**, 474.

Chest, Heart and Stroke Association (1982). Meeting on stroke units in the UK. Draft Report, eds Drs P. Blower, G. Mulley, and J.S. Watkins.

Chikos, P.M., Fisher, L.D., Hirsch, J.H., Harley, J.D., Thiele, B.L., and Strandness, D.E. (1983). Observer variability in evaluating extracranial carotid artery stenosis. *Stroke*, **14**, 885–92.

Chin, P., Angunawela, R., Mitchell, D., and Horne, J. (1980). Stroke register in Carlisle: a preliminary report. In *Clinical neuroepidemiology*, (ed. F.C. Rose), pp. 131–43. Pitman Medical, London.

Christie, D. (1981). Stroke in Melbourne, Australia: an epidemiological study. *Stroke*, **12**, 467–9.

Ciocon, J.O., Silverstone, F.A., Graver, L.M., and Foley, C.J. (1988). Tube feeding in elderly patients. Indications, benefits, and complications. *Archives of Internal Medicine*, **148**, 429–33.

Cochrane, A.L., Chapman, P.J., and Oldham, P.D. (1951). Observer errors in taking medical histories. *Lancet*, **1**, 1007–9.

Cohen, J. (1960). A coefficient of agreement for nominal scales. *Educational and Psychological Measurement*, **XX**, 37–46.

Cohn, J.N., Archibald, D.G., Ziesche, S. *et al.* (1986). Effect of vasodilator therapy on mortality in chronic congestive heart failure. *New England Journal of Medicine*, **314**, 1547–52.

Consensus Conference (1988). Treatment of stroke. *British Medical Journal*, **297**, 126–8.

Coope, J. and Warrender, T.S. (1986). Randomised trial of treatment of hypertension in elderly patients in primary care. *British Medical Journal*, **293**, 1145–8.

Cruickshank, J.M., Thorpe, J.M., and Zacharias, F.J. (1987). Benefits and potential harm of lowering high blood pressure. *Lancet*, **1**, 581–4; **2**, 695.

Cummins, R.O. (1983). Recent changes in salt use and stroke mortality in England & Wales. Any help for the salt-hypertension debate? *Journal of Epidemiology and Community Health*, **37**, 25–8.

Currie, C.T. (1986). Urinary incontinence after stroke. *British Medical Journal*, **293**, 1322–3.

David, R., Enderby, P., and Bainton, D. (1982). Treatment of acquired aphasia: speech therapists and volunteers compared. *Journal of Neurology, Neurosurgery and Psychiatry*, **45**, 957–61.

Dawber, T.R. (1980). The Framingham Study. London: Harvard University Press.

De Faire, U., Friberg, L., and Lundman, T. (1975). Concordance for mortality with special reference to ischaemic heart disease and cerebrovascular disease. *Preventive Medicine*, **4**, 509–17.

Dejong, G. and Branch, L.G. (1982). Predicting the stroke patient's ability to live independently. *Stroke*, **13**, 648–55.

Del Campo, C. (1988). Carotid endarterectomy trial: word of caution. *Lancet*, **1**, 1101–2.

Denham, M.J., Farran, H., and James, G. (1973). The value of 125-I-fibrinogen in the diagnosis of deep vein thrombosis in hemiplegia. *Age and Ageing*, **2**, 207–10.

Dennis, M.S., Bamford, J.M., Molyneux, A.J., and Warlow, C.P. (1987). Rapid resolution of signs of primary intracerebral haemorrhage in computed tomograms of the brain. *British Medical Journal*, **295**, 379–81.

Donaldson, S.W., Wagner, C.W., and Gresham, G.E. (1973). A unified ADL evaluation form. *Archives of Physical Medicine and Rehabilitation*, **54**, 175–80.

Droller, H. (1960). Survival after apoplexy. *Gerontology Clinics*, **2**, 120–8.

Dudley, H.A.F. (1987). Extracranial-intracranial bypass, one; clinical trials, nil. *British Medical Journal*, **294**, 1501–2.

Ebrahim, S. (1985) Physical disability, health, depressed mood, and use of services after stroke. Doctor of Medicine thesis, Nottingham University Medical School.

Ebrahim, S., Nouri, F., and Barer, D. (1985*a*). Cognitive failure after stroke. *Age and Ageing*, **14**, 345–8.

Ebrahim, S., Nouri, F., and Barer, D. (1985*b*). Measuring disability after a stroke. *Journal of Epidemiology and Community Health*, **39**, 86–9.

Ebrahim, S., Nouri, F., and Barer, D. (1986). Use of the Nottingham

Health Profile with patients after a stroke. *Journal of Epidemiology and Community Health*, **40**, 166–9.

Ebrahim, S. and Nouri, F. (1987) Carers of stroke patients. *International Rehabilitation Medicine*, **8**, 171–3.

Ebrahim, S., Nouri, F., and Barer, D. (1987*a*). Affective illness after stroke. *British Journal of Psychiatry*, **151**, 52–6.

Ebrahim, S., Barer, D., and Nouri, F. (1987*b*). An audit of follow-up services for stroke patients after discharge from hospital. *International Disability Studies*, **9**, 103–5.

Ebrahim, S., Dallosso, H., Morgan, K., Fentem, P., and Arie, T. (1988). Causes of ill-health in a random sample of old and very old people: prospects for prevention. *Journal of the Royal College of Physicians, London*, **22**, 105–7.

EC-IC Bypass Study Group (1985). Failure of extracranial arterial bypass to reduce the risk of ischaemic stroke. *New England Journal of Medicine*, **313**, 1191–1200.

Edmans, J.A. and Lincoln, N.B. (1989). Treatment of visual perceptual deficits after stroke: four single case studies. *International Disability Studies*, **11**, 25–33.

Eisenberg, H., Morrison, J.T., Sullivan, P., and Foote, F.M. (1964). Cerebrovascular accidents. Incidence and survival rates in a defined population, Middlesex County, Connecticut. *Journal of the American Medical Association*, **189**, 107–12.

Evans, J.G. (1979). The epidemiology of stroke. *Age and Ageing*, (*Suppl.*), **8**, 50–6.

Evans, J.G. (1987). Blood pressure and stroke in an elderly English population. *Journal of Epidemiology and Community Health*, **41**, 275–82.

Evans, J.G., Prudham, D., and Wandless, I. (1980). Risk factors for stroke in the elderly. In *The ageing brain. Neurological and mental disturbances*, (ed. G. Barbagallo and A.N. Exton-Smith), pp. 113–26. New York and London, Plenum Press.

Feldman, D.J., Lee, P.R., Unterecker, J. *et al.* (1962). A comparison of functionally orientated medical care and formal rehabilitation in the management of patients with hemiplegia due to cerebrovascular disease. *Journal of Chronic Diseases*, **15**, 297–310.

Field, D., Cordle, C.J., and Bowman, G.S. (1983). Coping with stroke at home. *International Rehabilitation Medicine*, **5**, 96–100.

Fields, W.S., Maslenikov, V., Meyer, J. *et al.* (1970). Joint study of extracranial arterial occlusion. V. Progress report of prognosis following surgery or non-surgical treatment for transient cerebral ischaemic attacks and cervical carotid artery lesions. *Journal of the American Medical Association*, **211**, 1993–2003.

Fisher, C.M. (1982). Disorientation for place. *Archives of Neurology*, **39**(1), 33–6.

Flegel, K.M., Shipley, M.J., and Rose, G. (1987). Risk of stroke in non-rheumatic atrial fibrillation. *Lancet*, **1**, 526–9.

Folstein, M.F., Folstein, S.E., and McHugh, P.R. (1975). Mini-Mental State. A practical method for grading the cognitive state of patients for the clinician. *Journal of Psychiatric Research*, **12**, 189–98.

Folstein, M.F., Maiberger, R., and McHugh, P.R. (1977). Mood disorder as a specific complication of stroke. *Journal of Neurology, Neurosurgery, and Psychiatry*, **40**, 1018–20.

Forfar, J.C. (1979). A 7 year analysis of haemorrhage in patients on long-term anticoagulant treatment. *British Heart Journal*, **42**, 128–32.

Forfar, J.C. (1982). Prediction of haemorrhage during long term oral coumarin anticoagulation by excessive prothrombin ratio. *American Heart Journal*, **103**, 445–6.

Freeling, P., Rao, B.M., Paykel, E.S., Sireling, L.I., and Burton, R.H. (1985). Unrecognised depression in general practice. *British Medical Journal*, **290**, 1880–3.

Freidman, R.C., Bigger, J.T., and Koranfield, D.S. (1971). The intern and sleep loss. *New England Journal of Medicine*, **285**, 201–3.

Garraway, M. and Akhtar, A.J. (1978). Theory and practice of stroke rehabilitation. In *Recent advances in geriatric medicine* (ed. B. Isaacs), pp. 7–20. Churchill Livingstone, London.

Garraway, W.M., Akhtar, A.J., Gore, S.M., Prescott, R.J., and Smith, R.G. (1976). Observer variation in the clinical assessment of stroke. *Age and Ageing*, **5**, 233–40.

Garraway, W.M., Whisnant, J.P., Furlan, A.J. *et al.* (1979). The declining incidence of stroke. *New England Journal of Medicine*, **300**, 449–52.

Garraway, W.M., Akhtar, A.J., Hockey, L., and Prescott, R.J. (1980*a*). Management of acute stroke in the elderly: preliminary results of a controlled trial. *British Medical Journal*, **280**, 1040–3.

Garraway, W.M., Akhtar, A.J., Hockey, L., and Prescott, R.J. (1980*b*). Management of acute stroke in the elderly: follow-up of a controlled trial. *British Medical Journal*, **281**, 827–9.

Garraway, W.M., Akhtar, A.J., Smith, D.L., and Smith, M.E. (1981). The triage of stroke rehabilitation. *Journal of Epidemiology and Community Health*, **35**, 39–44.

Garraway, W.M., Whisnant, J.P., and Drury, I. (1983*a*). The changing pattern of survival following stroke. *Stroke*, **14**, 699–703.

Garraway, W.M., Elverback, L.R., Connolly, D.C., and Whisnant, J.P. (1983*b*). The dichotomy of myocardial infarction and cerebral infarction. *Lancet*, **2**, 1332–5.

Gelmers, H.J., Gorter, K., de Weerdt, C.J., and Wiezer, H.J.A. (1988). A controlled trial of nimodopine in acute stroke. *New England Journal of Medicine*, **318**, 203–7.

Gennser, G., Rymark, P., and Isberg, P.E. (1988). Low birth weight and risk of high blood pressure in adulthood. *British Medical Journal*, **296**, 1498–1500.

Gent, M. (1987). Single studies and overview analyses: Is aspirin of value in cerebral ischemia? *Stroke*, **18**, 541–4.

Genton, E., Barnett, H., and Fields, W. (1977). Cerebral ischaemia: the role of thrombosis and antithrombotic therapy. *Stroke*, **8**, 150–75.

Gill, J.S., Zezulka, A.V., Shipley, M.J., Gill, S.K., and Beevers, D.G. (1986). Stroke and alcohol consumption. *New England Journal of Medicine*, **315**, 1041–6.

Glass, R., Allan, A., Uheinhuth, E., Kimball, C., and Borinstein, D. (1978). Psychiatric screening in a medical clinic. *Archives of General Psychiatry*, **35**, 1189–95.

Goble, R.E.A. (1976). Relevance of the ADL index. *British Journal of Occupational Therapy*, **39**, 12.

Goldberg, D. and Hillier, V. (1979). A scaled version of the General Health Questionnaire. *Psychological Medicine*, **9**, 139–45.

Goodwill, C.J. and Chamberlain, M.A. (ed.) (1988). *Rehabilitation of the physically disabled adult*. London, Croom Helm.

Gordon, C., Hewer, R.L., and Wade, D.T. (1987). Dysphagia in acute stroke. *British Medical Journal*, **295**, 411–14.

Gresham, G.E., Fitzpatrick, T.E., Wolf, P.A. *et al.* (1975). Residual disability in survivors of stroke—the Framingham study. *New England Journal of Medicine*, **293**, 954–6.

Gresham, G.E., Phillips, T.F., Wolf, P.A. *et al.* (1979). Epidemiological profile of long-term stroke disability: the Framingham study. *Archives of Physical Medicine and Rehabilitation*, **60**, 487–90.

Gresham, G.E., Phillips, T.F., and Labi, M.L.C. (1980). ADL status in stroke: relative merits of three standard indexes. *Archives of Physical Medicine and Rehabilitation*, **61**, 355–8.

Gross, C.R., Shinar, D., Mohr, J.P. *et al.* (1986). Interobserver agreement in the diagnosis of stroke type. *Archives of Neurology*, **43**, 893–8.

Gurling, H.M.D. (1984). Genetic epidemiology in medicine—recent twin research. *British Medical Journal*, **288**, 3–5.

Gurwitz, J.H., Goldberg, R.J., Holden, A., Knapie, N., and Ansell, J. (1988). Age-related risks of long-term anticoagulant therapy. *Archives of Internal Medicine*, **148**, 1733–6.

Haberman, S., Capildeo, R., and Rose, F.C. (1978). The changing mortality of cerebrovascular disease. *Quarterly Journal of Medicine*, **XLVII**, **185**, 71–88.

Haberman, S., Capildeo, R., and Rose, F.C. (1981). The seasonal variation in mortality from cerebrovascular disease. *Journal of Neurological Science*, **52**, 25–36.

Haberman, S., Capildeo, R., and Rose, F.C. (1982). Diverging trends in cerebrovascular disease and ischaemic heart disease mortality. *Stroke*, **13**, 582–9.

Hachinski, V.C., Lassen, N.A., and Marshall, J. (1985). Multi-infarct dementia, a cause of mental deterioration in the elderly. *Lancet*, **2**, 207–10.

Hachinski, V. (1986). Atrial fibrillation and recurrent stroke. *Archives of Neurology*, **43**, 70.

Haerer, A.F., Gotshall, R.A., Conneally, P.M. *et al.* (1977). Co-operative study of hospital frequency and character of transient ischemic attacks. *Journal of the American Medical Association*, **238**, 142–6.

Hampton, J. (1981). Presentation and analysis of the results of clinical trials in cardiovascular disease. *British Medical Journal*, **282**, 1371–3.

Hamrin, E. (1982*a*). Early activation in stroke: does it make a difference? *Scandinavian Journal of Rehabilitation Medicine*, **14**, 101–9.

Hamrin, E. (1982*b*). One year after stroke: a follow-up of an experimental study. *Scandinavian Journal of Rehabilitation Medicine*, **14**, 111–16.

Hanley, S., Bevan, J., Cockbill, S., and Heptinstall, S. (1981). Differential inhibition of low-dose aspirin of human venous prostacyclin synthesis and platelet thromboxane synthesis. *Lancet*, **1**, 969–71.

Harmsen, P. and Wilhelmsen, L. (1984). Stroke registration in Goteborg, Sweden, 1971–75. Clinical profile and prognosis. *Acta Medica Scandinavica*, **215**, 239–48.

Harrison, M.J.G. (1980). Clinical distinction of cerebral haemorrhage and infarction. *Postgraduate Medical Journal*, **56**, 629–32.

Harrison, M. (1984). Hypertension and stroke. *British Journal of Hospital Medicine*, **31**, 215–18.

Hatano, S. (1976) Experience from a multicentre stroke register: a preliminary report. *Bulletin of the World Health Organization*, **54**, 541–53.

Havlik, R.J., Garrison, R.J., Feinleb, M. *et al.* (1979). Blood pressure aggregation in families. *American Journal of Epidemiology*, **110**, 304–12.

Hawton, K. (1981). The long term outcome of psychiatric morbidity detected in general medical patients. *Journal of Psychosomatic Research*, **25**, 237–43.

Heasman, M.A. and Lipworth, L. (1966). Accuracy of certification of cause of death. *Studies on Medical and Population Subjects*, No. 20, pp. 23–4. HMSO, London.

Heller, A., Wade, D.T., Wood, V.A. *et al.* (1987). Arm function after stroke: measurement and recovery over the first three months. *Journal of Neurology, Neurosurgery, and Psychiatry*, **50**, 714–19.

Henley, S., Pettit, S., Todd-Pokropek, A., and Tupper, A. (1985). Who goes home? Predictive factors in stroke recovery. *Journal of Neurology, Neurosurgery, and Psychiatry*, **48**, 1–6.

Herman, B., Schulte, B.P.M., Van Luijk, J.H., Leyten, A.C.M., and Frenken, C.W.G.M. (1980). Epidemiology of stroke in Tilburg, The Netherlands. The population-based stroke incidence register:1. Introduction and preliminary results. *Stroke*, **11**, 162–5.

Herman, B., Leyeten, A.C.M., Van Luijk, J.H. *et al.* (1982*a*). Epidemiology of stroke in Tilburg, The Netherlands. The population-based stroke incidence register:2. Incidence, initial clinical picture and medical care, and three-week case fatality. *Stroke*, **13**, 629–34.

Herman, B., Leyten, A.C.M., Van Luijk, J.H. *et al.* (1982*b*). An evaluation of risk factors for stroke in a Dutch community. *Stroke*, **13**, 334–9.

Herman, B., Schmitz, P.I.M., Leyten, A.C.M. *et al.* (1983). Multivariate logistic analysis of the risk factors for stroke in Tilburg, The Netherlands. *American Journal of Epidemiology*, **118**, 514–25.

Hewer, R.L. (1987). Dysphagia after stroke. *British Medical Journal*, **295**, 1137.

Heyman, A., Wilkinson, E.E., and Hurwitz, B.J. *et al.* (1984). Risk of ischaemic heart disease in patients with TIA. *Neurology*, **34**, 626–30.

Hill, A.B. (1965). The environment and disease: association or causation. *Proceedings of the Royal Society of Medicine*, **58**, 295–300.

Hill, A.B., Marshall, J., and Shaw, D. (1962). Cerebrovascular disease: trial of long term anticoagulant therapy. *British Medical Journal*, **2**, 1003–5.

Hillbohm, M. and Kaste, M. (1983). Ethanol intoxication: a risk factor for ischaemic brain infarction. *Stroke*, **14**, 694–9.

Hilton, P. and Stanton, S. (1981). Algorithmic method for assessing urinary incontinence in elderly women. *British Medical Journal*, **282**, 940–2.

Himmelmann, A., Hansson, L., Svensson, A. *et al.* (1988). Predictors of stroke in the elderly. *Acta Medica Scandinavica*, **224**, 439–43.

Hodkinson, H.M. (1972). Evaluation of a mental test score for assessment of mental impairment in the elderly. *Age and Ageing*, **1**, 233–8.

Hopkins, A. (1975). The need for speech therapy for dysphasia following stroke. *Health Trends*, **7**, 58–60.

House, A. (1987). Depression after stroke. *British Medical Journal*, **294**, 76–8.

House, A., Dennis, M., Molyneux, A., Warlow, C., and Hawton, K. (1989). Emotionalism after stroke. *British Medical Journal*, **298**, 991–4.

Howard, D. (1984). Speech therapy for aphasic stroke patients. *Lancet*, **1**, 1413–14.

Hunt, S., McEwan, J., and McKenna, S. (1986). Measuring health status. Croom Helm, London.

Hurwitz, L.J. and Adams, G.F. (1972). Rehabilitation of hemiplegia: indices of assessment and prognosis. *British Medical Journal*, **1**, 94–8.

Hypertension Detection and Follow-up Program (1979). Five year findings of the HDFP. 1. Reduction in mortality of persons with high blood pressure, including mild hypertension. *Journal of the American Medical Association*, **242**, 2562–71, 2572–7.

Hypertension Stroke Cooperative Study Group (1974). Effect of antihypertensive treatment on stroke recurrence. *Journal of the American Medical Association*, **229**, 409–18.

International Multicentre Trial (1975). Prevention of postoperative pulmonary emboli by low doses of heparin. *Lancet*, **2**, 45–51.

Intersalt Cooperative Research Group (1988). Intersalt: an international study of electrolyte excretion and blood pressure. Results for 24 hour urinary sodium and potassium excretion. *British Medical Journal*, **297**, 319–28.

Isaacs, B. (1971). Identification of disability in the stroke patient. *Modern Geriatrics*, **1**, 390–402.

Isaacs, B. and Marks, R. (1973). Determinants of outcome of stroke rehabilitation. *Age and Ageing*, **2**, 139–49.

Isaacs, B., Neville, Y., and Rushford, I. (1976). The stricken: the social consequences of stroke. *Age and Ageing*, **2**, 139–49.

Italian Acute Stroke Study Group (1988). Haemodilution in acute stroke: results of the Italian haemodilution trial. *Lancet*, **1**, 318–21.

Jansen, P., Schulte, B., Meyboom, R., and Gribnau, F. (1986*a*). Antihypertensive treatment as a possible cause of strokes in the elderly. *Age and Ageing*, **15**, 129–38.

Jansen, P., Gribnau, F., Schulte, B., and Poels, E. (1986*b*). Contribution of inappropriate treatment for hypertension to pathogenesis of stroke in the elderly. *British Medical Journal*, **293**, 914–17.

Jarvik, L.F. and Matsuyama, S.S. (1983). Parental stroke: risk factor for multi-infarct dementia? *Lancet*, **2**, 1025.

Jay, P. (1976). How the association sought a standard way to record assessment. *British Journal of Occupational Therapy*, **39**, 36.

Johnston, J., Beevers, D., Dunn, F., Larkin, H., and Titterington, D. (1981). The importance of good blood pressure control in the prevention of stroke recurrence in hypertensive patients. *Postgraduate Medical Journal*, **57**, 690–3.

Jones, D. and Vetter, N.J. (1985). Formal and informal support received by carers of elderly dependants. *British Medical Journal*, **291**, 643–5.

Joosens, J.V., Kestelloot, H., and Amery, A. (1979). Salt intake and mortality from stroke. *New England Journal of Medicine*, **300**, 1396.

Kagan, A., Yano, K., Rhoads, G. *et al.* (1979). Is the reported high mortality from cerebrovascular disease in Japan really an artifact? *Journal of Chronic Diseases*, **32**, 153–6.

Kannel, W.B. and Wolf, P.A. (1983). Epidemiology of cerebrovascular disease. In *Vascular disease of the central nervous system*, (ed. R.W. Ross Russell) (2nd edn) pp. 1–24. Churchill Livingstone, Edinburgh.

Kannel, W.B., Gordon, T., Wolf, P.A., and McNamara, P. (1972). Haemoglobin and the risk of cerebral infarction. The Framingham study. *Stroke*, **3**, 409–20.

Kannel, W.B., Wolf, P.A., and Verter, J. (1983). Manifestations of coronary disease predisposing to stroke. The Framingham study. *Journal of the American Medical Association*, **250**, 2942–6.

Katz, S., Ford, A.B., Moskowitz, R.W., Jackson, B.A., and Jaffe, W. (1963). Studies of illness in the aged. The index of ADL: a standardised measure of biological and psychosocial function. *Journal of the American Medical Association*, **185**, 914–19.

Keatinge, W.R. (1986). Seasonal mortality among elderly people with unrestricted home heating. *British Medical Journal*, **293**, 732–3.

Keatinge, W.R., Coleshaw, S.R.K., Cotter, F. *et al.* (1984). Increases in platelet and red cell counts, blood viscosity, and arterial pressure during mild surface cooling: factors in mortality from coronary and cerebral thrombosis in winter. *British Medical Journal*, **289**, 1405–8.

Kelman, H.R. and Willner, A. (1962). Problems of measurement and evaluation in rehabilitation. *Archives of Physical Medicine and Rehabilitation*, **4**, 172–81.

Khaw, K.T. and Barrett-Connor, E. (1986). Family history of stroke as an independent predictor of ischaemic heart disease in men and stroke in women. *American Journal of Epidemiology*, **123**, 59–66.

Khaw, K.T. and Barrett-Connor, E. (1987). Dietary potassium and stroke associated mortality. A 12-year prospective population study. *New England Journal of Medicine*, **316**, 235–40.

Kinsella, G. and Ford, B. (1985). Hemi-inattention and the recovery patterns of stroke patients. *International Rehabilitation Medicine*, **7**, 102–6.

Klatsky, A.L., Freidman, G.D., Siegelaub, A.B., and Gerard, M.J. (1977). Alcohol consumption and blood pressure. Kaiser-Permanente Multiphasic Health Examination Data. *New England Journal of Medicine*, **296**, 1194–1200.

Knights, E., and Folstein, M.F. (1977). Unsuspected emotional and cognitive disturbance in medical patients. *Annals of Internal Medicine*, **87**, 723–4.

Knox, E.G. (1981). Meteorological associations of cerebrovascular disease mortality in England and Wales. *Journal of Epidemiology and Community Health*, **35**, 220–3.

Kotila, M. (1984). Declining incidence and mortality of stroke? *Stroke*, **15**, 255–9.

Kotila, M., Waltimo, O., Niemi, M.L., Laaksonen, R., and Lempinen, M. (1984). The profile of recovery from stroke and factors influencing outcome. *Stroke*, **15**, 1039–44.

Kotila, M., Waltimo, O., Niemi, M.L., and Laaksonen, R. (1986*a*). Dementia after stroke. *European Neurology*, **25**, 134–40.

Kotila, M., Niemi, M.L., and Laaksonen, R. (1986*b*). Four-year prognosis of stroke patients with visuospatial inattention. *Scandinavian Journal of Rehabilitation Medicine*, **18**, 177–9.

Koudstaal, P.J., Stibbe, J., and Vermeulen, M. (1988). Fatal ischaemic brain oedema after early thrombolysis with tissue plasminogen activator in acute stroke. *British Medical Journal*, **297**, 1571–4.

Landis, J.R. and Koch, G.G. (1977). The measurement of observer agreement for categorical data. *Biometrics*, **33**, 159–74.

Langton-Hewer, R. (1973). Stroke rehabilitation: some current problems. *Proceedings of the Royal Society of Medicine*, **66**, 882–4.

Lee, M.C., Heaney, L.M., Jacobson, R.L., and Klassen, A.C. (1975). Cerebrospinal fluid in cerebral haemorrhage and infarction. *Stroke*, **6**, 638–41.

Legh-Smith, J.A., Denis, R., Enderby, P., Wade, D.T., and Hewer, R.L. (1987). Selection of aphasic stroke patients for intensive speech therapy. *Journal of Neurology, Neurosurgery, and Psychiatry*, **50**, 1488–92.

Lendrum, W. and Lincoln, N.B. (1985). Spontaneous recovery of language in patients with aphasia between 4 and 34 weeks after stroke. *Journal of Neurology, Neurosurgery, and Psychiatry*, **48**, 743–8.

Lincoln, N.B., McGuirk, E., Mulley, G.P. *et al.* (1984). Effectiveness of speech therapy for aphasic stroke patients. *Lancet*, **1**, 1197–1200.

Lipsey, J.R., Robinson, R.G., Pearlson, G.D., Rao, K., and Price, T.R. (1984). Nortriptyline treatment of post-stroke depression: a double blind study. *Lancet*, **1**, 297–300.

Lipsey, J.R., Robinson, R.G., Pearlson, G.D., Rao, K., and Price, T.R. (1985). The dexamethasone suppression test and mood following stroke. *American Journal of Psychiatry*, **142**, 318–23.

Lodder, J., Dennis, M.S., Van Raak, L., Jones, L.N., and Warlow, C.P. (1988). Cooperative study on the value of long term anticoagulation in patients with stroke and non-rheumatic atrial fibrillation. *British Medical Journal*, **296**, 1435–8.

Loftus, C.M., Biller, J., Godersky, J.C. *et al.* (1988). Carotid endarterectomy in symptomatic elderly patients. *Neurosurgery*, **22**, 676–80.

Lorenze, E.J., Simon, H., and Linden, J. (1959). Urological problems in the rehabilitation of hemiplegic patients. *Journal of the American Medical Association*, **169**, 1042–6.

Lowe, G.D.O., Jaap, A.J., and Forbes, C.D. (1983). Relation of atrial fibrillation and high haematocrit to mortality in acute stroke. *Lancet*, **1**, 784–6.

McAvoy, B.R. (1986). Death after bereavement. *British Medical Journal*, **293**, 835–6.

MacGuire, G., Julier, D., Hawton, K., and Bancroft, J. (1974). Psychiatric morbidity and referral in two general medical wards. *British Medical Journal*, **1**, 268–70.

McCarthy, S.T. and Turner, J.J. (1986). Low dose subcutaneous heparin in the prevention of deep vein thrombosis and pulmonary emboli following acute stroke. *Age and Ageing*, **15**, 84–8.

McCarthy, S.T., Turner, J.J., Robertson, D., Hawkey, C.J., and Macey, D.J. (1977). Low dose heparin after acute stroke. *Lancet*, **2**, 800–1.

Mahoney, F.I. and Barthel, D.W. (1965). Functional evaluation: the Barthel Index. *Maryland State Medical Journal*, **14**, 61–5.

Malmgren, R., Warlow, C., Bamford, J., and Sandercock, P. (1987). Geographical and secular trends in stroke incidence. *Lancet*, **2**, 1196–9.

Marshall, J. and Shaw, D.A. (1959). The natural history of cerebrovascular disease. *British Medical Journal*, **1**, 1614–17.

Marquardsen, J. (1969). *The natural history of acute cerebrovascular disease*. Munksgaard, Copenhagen.

Martin, J.F., Hamdy, N., Nicholl, J. *et al.* (1985). Double-blind controlled trial of prostacyclin in cerebral infarction. *Stroke*, **16**, 386–90.

Matsumoto, N., Whisnant, J.P., Kurland, L.T., and Okazaki, H. (1973). Natural history of stroke in Rochester, Minnesota, 1955 through 1969: an extension of a previous study, 1945 through 1954. *Stroke*, **4**, 20–9.

Mattilla, K., Haavisto, M., Rajala, S., and Heikinheimo, R. (1988). Blood pressure and survival in the very old. *British Medical Journal*, **296**, 887–9.

MRC (Medical Research Council) Working Party (1985). MRC trial of treatment of mild hypertension: principal results. *British Medical Journal*, **291**, 97–104.

MRC (Medical Research Council) Working Party (1988). Stroke and coronary heart disease in mild hypertension: risk factors and the value of treatment. *British Medical Journal*, **296**, 1565–70.

Meade, T.W. (1977). Problems for the research worker in rehabilitation studies. *Rheumatology and Rehabilitation*, **16**, 254–6.

Meade, T.W., Gardner, M.J., Cannon, P. *et al.* (1968). Observer variability in the recording of peripheral pulses. *British Heart Journal*, **30**, 661–5.

Merrett, J.D. and Adams, G.F. (1966). Comparison of mortality rates in elderly hypertensive and normotensive hemiplegic patients. *British Medical Journal*, **2**, 802–5.

Meikle, M., Wechsler, E., Tupper, A. *et al.* (1979). Comparative trial of volunteer and professional treatments of dysphasia after stroke. *British Medical Journal*, **2**, 87–9.

Meissner, I., Whisnant, J.P., and Garraway, W.M. (1988). Hypertension management and stroke recurrence in a community (Rochester, Minnesota), 1950–1979. *Stroke*, **19**, 459–63.

Miall, W.E. and Oldham, P.D. (1963). The hereditary factor in arterial blood pressure. *British Medical Journal*, **1**, 75–80.

Miall, W.E., Henage, P., Kholsa, T., Lovell, H.G., and Moore, F. (1967). Factors influencing the degree of resemblance in arterial pressure of close relatives. *Clinical Science*, **33**, 271–83.

Michaels, J.A. (1988). Surgical audit and carotid endarterectomy. *Lancet*, **2**, 110–11.

Mills, D.C. and Smith, J.B. (1972). The control of platelet responsiveness by agents that influence cyclic AMP levels. *Annals of the New York Academy of Sciences*, **210**, 391–9.

Mitchell, J.R.A. (1982). But will it help my patients with infarction? The implications of recent trials for everyday country folk. *British Medical Journal*, **285**, 1140–8.

Mulley, G.P. (1982). Avoidable complications of stroke. *Journal of the Royal College of Physicians, London*, **16**, 94–7.

Mulley, G.P., Wilcock, R.G., and Mitchell, J.R.A. (1978). Dexamethasone in acute stroke. *British Medical Journal*, **2**, 994–6.

Murphy, E. (1982). Social origins of depression in old age. *British Journal of Psychiatry*, **141**, 135–42.

Nabarro, J. (1984). Unrecognised psychiatric illness in medical patients. *British Medical Journal*, **289**, 635–6.

Newman, G. and Mitchell, J.R.A. (1984). Homocystinuria presenting as multiple arterial occlusions. *Quarterly Journal of Medicine*, **LIII**, 251–8.

Nicholls, E.S. and Johansen, H.L. (1983). Implications of the changing trends in cerebrovascular and ischemic heart disease mortality. *Stroke*, **14**, 153–5.

Norris, J.W. and Hachinski, V.C. (1982). Misdiagnosis of stroke. *Lancet*, **1**, 328–31.

O'Brien, J.R. (1980). Platelets and vessel wall. How much aspirin? *Lancet*, **1**, 372–3.

O'Brien, P.A., Ryder, D.Q., and Twomey, C. (1987). The role of computed tomographic brain scans in the diagnosis of acute stroke in the elderly. *Age and Ageing*, **16**, 319–22.

Ostfeld, A.M. (1980). A review of stroke epidemiology. *Epidemiologic Reviews*, **2**, 136–52.

Oxbury, J.M., Greenhall, R.C.D., and Grainger, K.M.R. (1975). Predicting the outcome of stroke: acute stage after cerebral infarction. *British Medical Journal*, **3**, 125–7.

Oxfordshire Community Stroke Project (1983). Incidence of stroke in Oxfordshire: first year's experience of a community stroke register. *British Medical Journal*, **287**, 713–17.

Paganini-Hill, A., Ross, R.K., and Henderson, B.E. (1988). Postmenopausal oestrogen treatment and stroke: a prospective study. *British Medical Journal*, **297**, 519–21.

Partridge, C.J., Johnston, M., and Edwards, S. (1987). Recovery from physical disability after stroke: normal patterns as a basis for evaluation. *Lancet*, **1**, 373–5.

Pearson, T.C. and Wetherley-Mein, G. (1978). Vascular occlusive episodes and venous haematocrit in primary proliferative polycythaemia. *Lancet*, **2**, 1219–22.

Peto, R. (1978). Clinical trial methodology. *Biomedicine* (Special Issue), **28**, 24–36.

Peto, R. (1982). Long term and short term beta-blockade after myocardial infarction. *Lancet*, **1**, 1159–61.

Peto, R., Pike, M.C., Armitage, P. *et al.* (1976). Design and analysis of randomised clinical trials requiring prolonged observation of each patient. I. *British Journal of Cancer*, **34**, 585–612.

Peto, R., Pike, M.C., Armitage, P. *et al.* (1977). Design and analysis of randomised clinical trials requiring prolonged observation of each patient. II. *British Journal of Cancer*, **35**, 1–39.

Power, M.J., Fullerton, K.J., and Stout, R.W. (1988). Blood glucose and prognosis of acute stroke. *Age and Ageing*, **17**, 164–70.

Prescott, R.J., Garraway, W.M., and Akhtar, A.J. (1982). Predicting functional outcome following acute stroke using a standard clinical examination. *Stroke*, **13**, 641–7.

Rankin, J. (1957). Cerebral vascular accidents in patients over the age of 60: II. Prognosis. *Scottish Medical Journal*, **2**, 200–15.

Redding, M.J., Orto, L.A., Winter, S.W. *et al.* (1986). Antidepressant therapy after stroke. A double-blind trial. *Archives of Neurology*, **43**, 763–5.

Ritchie, K. (1988). The screening of cognitive impairment in the elderly. *Journal of Clinical Epidemiology*, **41**, 635–43.

Robinson, R.G. and Price, T.R. (1982). Post stroke depressive disorders: a follow up study of 103 patients. *Stroke*, **13**, 635–41.

Robinson, R.G., Starr, L.B., and Price, T.R. (1984*a*). A two year longitudinal study of mood disorder following stroke: prevalence and duration at six months follow up. *British Journal of Psychiatry*, **144**, 256–62.

Robinson, R.G., Kubos, K.L., Starr, L.B., Rao, K., and Price, T.R. (1984*b*). Mood disorders in stroke patients. Importance of location of lesion. *Brain*, **107**, 81–93.

Robinson, R.G., Bolla-Wilson, K., Kaplan, E., Lipsey, J., and Price, T.R. (1986). Depression influences intellectual impairment in stroke patients. *British Journal of Psychiatry*, **148**, 541–7.

Roos, J. and van Roost, H.E. (1965). The cause of bleeding during anticoagulant treatment. *Acta Medica Scandinavica*, **178**, 129–31.

Rose, G. (1981). Strategy of prevention: lessons from cardiovascular disease. *British Medical Journal*, **280**, 1847–51.

Royal College of Physicians, London (1974). *Report of Geriatrics Committee Working Group on Strokes*. London.

Ruff, R.L. and Dougherty, J.H. (1981). Evaluation of acute cerebral ischaemia for anticoagulant therapy: computed tomography or lumbar puncture. *Neurology*, **31**, 736–40.

Sacco, R., Wolf, P., Kannel, W., and McNamara, P. (1982). Survival and recurrence following stroke. The Framingham Study. *Stroke*, **13**, 290–5.

Sackett, D., Haynes, R.B., and Tugwell, P. (1985). *Clinical epidemiology: A basic science for clinical medicine*. Little, Brown & Co, Boston and Toronto.

Sacquegna, T., deCarolis, P., Andreoli, A. *et al.* (1984). Long term prognosis after occlusion of the middle cerebral artery. *British Medical Journal*, **288**, 1490–1.

Safar, P. (1980). Amelioration of post-ischemic brain damage with barbiturates. *Stroke*, **11**, 565–8.

Sage, J. and Van Uitert, R. (1983). Risk of recurrent stroke in patients with atrial fibrillation and non-valvular heart disease. *Stroke*, **14**, 537–40.

Sainsbury, S. (1973). *Measuring disability*. Occasional Papers in Social Administration. No. 54, pp. 35–62. Bell, London.

Salonen, J.T., Puska, P., Tuomilheto, J., and Homan, K. (1982). Relation of blood pressure, serum lipids, and smoking to the risk of cerebral stroke. *Stroke*, **13**, 327–33.

Sandercock, P. (1987*a*). Asymptomatic carotid stenosis: spare the knife. *British Medical Journal*, **294**, 1368–9.
Sandercock, P. (1987*b*). Important new treatments for acute ischaemic stroke? *British Medical Journal*, **295**, 1224–5.
Sandercock, P. and Warlow, C. (1985). The prevention of stroke in the elderly. In *Prevention of disease in the elderly*, (ed. J.A.M. Gray), pp. 130–55. Churchill Livingstone, London.
Sandercock, P., Molyneux, A., and Warlow, C. (1985*a*). The value of CT scanning in patients with stroke: Oxford Community Stroke Project. *British Medical Journal*, **290**, 193–6.
Sandercock, P., Allen, C., Corston, R., Harrison, M.J.G., and Warlow, C.P. (1985*b*). Clinical diagnosis of intracranial haemorrhage using Guy's Hospital score. *British Medical Journal*, **291**, 1675–7.
Sandercock, P., Warlow, C., Bamford, J., Peto, R., and Starkey, I. (1986). Is a controlled trial of long-term anticoagulants in patients with stroke and non-rheumatic atrial fibrillation worthwhile? *Lancet*, **1**, 788–92.
Sandercock, P., Warlow, C.P., Jones, L.N., and Starkey, I.R. (1989). Predisposing factors for cerebral infarction: the Oxfordshire community stroke project. *British Medical Journal*, **298**, 75–80.
Sartwell, P.E. and Stolley, P.D. (1982). Oral contraceptives and vascular disease. *Epidemiologic Reviews*, **4**, 95–109.
Saunders, J.B. (1987). Alcohol: an important cause of hypertension. *British Medical Journal*, **294**, 1045–6.
Scandinavian Stroke Study Group (1987). Multicentre trial of hemodilution in acute ischaemic stroke. I. Results in the total patient population. *Stroke*, **18**, 691–9.
Scandinavian Stroke Study Group (1988). Multicentre trial of hemodilution in acute ischaemic stroke. Results of subgroup analyses. *Stroke*, **19**, 464–71.
Schwartz, D. and Lellouch, J. (1967). Explanatory and pragmatic attitudes in therapeutic trials. *Journal of Chronic Diseases*, **20**, 637–48.
Scmidt, E.V., Smirnov, V.E., and Ryabova, V.S. (1988). Results of the seven-year prospective study of stroke patients. *Stroke*, **19**, 942–9.
Seale, C. and Davies, P. (1987). Outcome measurement in stroke rehabilitation. *International Disability Studies*, **9**, 155–60.
Selley, W.G. (1985). Swallowing difficulties in stroke patients: a new treatment. *Age and Ageing*, **14**, 361–5.
Shaw, D.A., Venables, G.S., Cartlidge, N.E.F., Bates, D., and Dickinson, P.H. (1984). Carotid endarterectomy in patients with transient cerebral ischaemia. *Journal of Neurological Science*, **64**, 45–53.
Sheikh, K., Smith, D.S., Meade, T.W. *et al.* (1979). Repeatability and validity of a modified ADL index in studies of chronic disability. *International Journal of Rehabilitation Medicine*, **1**, 51–8.
Sheikh, K., Brennan, P.J., Meade, T.W., Smith, D.S., and Goldenberg, E.

(1983). Predictors of mortality and disability in stroke. *Journal of Epidemiology and Community Health*, **37**, 70–4.

Sherman, D.G., Hart, R., and Easton, J.D. (1986). The secondary prevention of stroke in patients with atrial fibrillation. *Archives of Neurology*, **43**, 68–70.

Shinar, D., Gross, C.R., Mohr, J.P. *et al.* (1985). Interobserver variability in the assessment of neurologic history and examination in the stroke data bank. *Archives of Neurology*, **42**, 557–65.

Shinar, D., Gross, C.R., Hier, D.B. *et al.* (1987). Interobserver reliability in the interpretation of computed tomographic scans of stroke patients. *Archives of Neurology*, **44**, 149–55.

Sigurdsson, G., Sigfusson, N., Thorsteinsson, T. *et al.* (1983). Screening for health risks. How useful is a questionnaire response showing a family history of myocardial infarction, hypertension, or stroke? *Acta Medica Scandinavica*, **213**, 45–50.

Sila, C.A. and Furlan, A.J. (1988). Drug treatment of stroke. Current status and future prospects. *Drugs*, **35**, 468–76.

Simpson, F.O. (1979). Salt and hypertension: a sceptical review of the evidence. *Clinical Science*, **57**, 463s–80s.

Sinyor, D., Amato, P., Kalonpek, D.G., Becker, R., Goldenberg, M., and Coopersmith, H. (1986). Post-stroke depression and lesion location: an attempted replication. *Brain*, **109**, 537–46.

Sixty-plus Reinfarction Study Research Group (1980). A double-blind trial to assess long-term oral anticoagulant therapy in elderly patients after myocardial infarction. *Lancet*, **2**, 989–94.

Sixty-plus Reinfarction Study Research Group (1982). Risks of long-term oral anticoagulant therapy in elderly patients after myocardial infarction. *Lancet*, **1**, 64–8.

Skilbeck, C.E., Wade, D.T., Hewer, R.L., and Wood, V.A. (1983). Recovery after stroke. *Journal of Neurology, Neurosurgery, and Psychiatry*, **46**, 5–8.

Sloan, M.A. (1987). Thrombolysis and stroke. Past and future. *Archives of Neurology*, **44**, 748–68.

Smith, D.S., Goldenberg, E., Ashburn, A. *et al.* (1981). Remedial therapy after stroke: a randomised controlled trial. *British Medical Journal*, **282**, 517–20.

Sox, H.C., Blatt, M.A., Higgins, M.C., and Marton, K.I. (1988). *Medical decision making*. Butterworths, London.

Spiteri, M.A., Cook, D.G., and Clarke, S.W. (1988). Reliability of eliciting physical signs in the examination of the chest. *Lancet*, **1**, 873–5.

Spranger, M., Aspey, B.S., and Harrison, M.J.G. (1989). Sex difference in antithrombotic effect of aspirin. *Stroke*, **20**, 34–7.

Stamp, E., Jones, S., Ryrie, D., and Hedley, A.J. (1985). Oral anticoagulants: a cost effectiveness approach. *Journal of the Royal College of Physicians, London*, **19**, 105–8.

Starkey, I. and Warlow, C. (1986). The secondary prevention of stroke in patients with atrial fibrillation. *Archives of Neurology*, **43**, 66–8.

Stein, R.E.K., Gortmaker, S.L., Perrin, E.C. *et al.* (1987). Severity of illness: concepts and measurements. *Lancet*, **2**, 1506–9.

Steiner, T.J. (1989). Fatal ischaemic brain oedema after tissue plasminogen activator. *British Medical Journal*, **298**, 382.

Steiner, T.J. and Rose, F.C. (1986). Towards a model stroke trial. The single-centre Naftidrofuryl Study. *Neuroepidemiology*, **5**, 121–47.

Stevens, R. and Ambler, N. (1982). The incidence and survival of stroke patients in a defined community. *Age and Ageing*, **11**, 266–74.

Stevens, R., Ambler, N.R., and Warren, M.D. (1984). A randomized controlled trial of a stroke rehabilitation ward. *Age and Ageing*, **13**, 65–75.

Stone, S.P. (1987). The Mount Vernon stroke service: a feasibility study to determine whether it is possible to apply the principles of stroke unit management to patients and their families on general medical wards. *Age and Ageing*, **16**, 81–8.

Strand, T., Asplund, K., Erikkson, S. *et al.* (1984). A randomized controlled trial of hemodilution therapy in acute ischaemic stroke. *Stroke*, **15**, 980–9.

Sunderland, A., Wade, D.T., and Hewer, R.L. (1987). The natural history of visual neglect after stroke. Indications from two methods of assessment. *International Disability Studies*, **9**, 55–9.

Svanborg, A. (1988). The health of the elderly population: results from longitudinal studies with age-cohort comparisons. In *Research and the ageing population* (ed. D. Evered and J. Whelan), pp. 3–16. John Wiley, Chichester.

Swets, J.A., Pickett, R.M., Whitehead, S.F. *et al.* (1979). Assessment of diagnostic technologies. *Science*, **205**, 753–9.

Syrjanen, J., Valtonen, V.V., Iivanainen, M., Kaste, M., and Huttunen, J.K. (1988). Preceding infection as an important risk factor for ischaemic brain infarction in young and middle aged patients. *British Medical Journal*, **296**, 1156–60.

Sze, P.C., Reitman, D., Pincus, M.M., Sacks, H.S., and Chalmers, T.C. (1988). Antiplatelet agents in the secondary prevention of stroke: meta-analysis of the randomized control trials. *Stroke*, **19**, 436–42.

Tanaka, H., Ueda, Y., Date, C. *et al.* (1981). Incidence of stroke in Shibata, Japan: 1976–1978. *Stroke*, **12**, 460–6.

Tanaka, H., Ueda, Y., Hayashi, M. *et al.* (1982). Risk factors for cerebral haemorrhage and cerebral infarction in a Japanese rural community. *Stroke*, **13**, 62–73.

Tapp, A., Fall, M., Norgaard, J. *et al.* (1987). A dose titrated, multicentre study of terodiline in the treatment of detrusor instability. *Neurology and Urodynamics*, **6**, 254–5.

Thomas, D.J. (1984). Treatment of acute stroke. *British Medical Journal*, **288**, 2–3.

Tinson, D.J. and Lincoln, N.B. (1987). Subjective memory impairment after stroke. *International Disability Studies*, **9**, 6–9.

Tohgi, H., Yamanouchi, H., Murakami, M., and Kameyama, M. (1978). Importance of the hematocrit as a risk factor in cerebral infarction. *Stroke*, **9**, 369–74.

Tohgi, H., Mochizuki, H., Yamanouchi, H. *et al.* (1981). A comparison between the computed tomogram and neuropathological findings in cerebrovascular disease. *Journal of Neurology*, **224**, 211–20.

Tomasello, F., Mariani, F., Fieschi, C. *et al.* (1982). Assessment of inter-observer differences in the Italian multicenter study on reversible cerebral ischaemia. *Stroke*, **13**, 32–5.

Tomlinson, B.E., Blessed, G., and Roth, M. (1970). Observations on the brains of demented old people. *Journal of Neurological Science*, **11**, 205–42.

Toumilehto, J., Nissinen, A., Wold, E. *et al.* (1985). Effectiveness of treatment with antihypertensive drugs and trends in mortality from stroke in the community. *British Medical Journal*, **291**, 857–60.

Toumilehto, J., Geboers, J., Salonen, J.T. *et al.* (1986). Decline in cardio-vascular mortality in North Karelia and other parts of Finland. *British Medical Journal*, **293**, 1068–71.

Townsend, J., Piper, M., Frank, A.O. *et al.* (1988). Reduction in hospital readmission stay of elderly patients by a community based discharge scheme: a randomised controlled trial. *British Medical Journal*, **297**, 544–7.

Ueda, K., Omae, T., Hirota, Y. *et al.* (1981). Decreasing trend in incidence and mortality from stroke in Hisayama Residents, Japan. *Stroke*, **12**, 154–60.

UK-TIA Study Group (1979). Design and protocol of the UK-TIA aspirin study. In *Drug treatment and prevention in cerebrovascular disorders* (ed. G. Tognoni and S. Garattini), pp. 387–94. Elsevier, Amsterdam.

UK-TIA Study Group (1983). Variation in the use of angiography and carotid endarterectomy by neurologists in the UK-TIA aspirin trial. *British Medical Journal*, **286**, 514–17.

UK-TIA Study Group (1988). United Kingdom transient ischaemic attack (UK-TIA) aspirin trial: interim results. *British Medical Journal*, **296**, 316–20.

Vandenbroucke, J.P. (1988). Passive smoking and lung cancer: a publication bias? *British Medical Journal*, **296**, 391–2.

Veterans Administration Cooperative Study Group on Antihypertensive Agents (1970). Effects of treatment on morbidity in hypertension. II. Results in patients with diastolic blood pressures averaging 90 through 114 mmHg. *Journal of the American Medical Association*, **213**, 1143–52.

Viitanen, M., Winblad, B., and Asplund, K. (1987). Autopsy-verified causes of death after stroke. *Acta Medica Scandinavica*, **222**, 401–8.

von Arbin, M., Britton, M., De Faire, U. *et al.* (1981). Accuracy of bedside diagnosis of stroke. *Stroke*, **12**, 288–93.

Wade, D.T. (1986). Stroke assessment: it's time we all spoke the same language. *Geriatric Medicine*, **16**, 11–12.

Wade, D.T. and Collin, C. (1988). The Barthel ADL Index: a standard measure of physical disability. *International Disability Studies*, **10**, 64–7.

Wade, D.T. and Hewer, R.L. (1985*a*). Outlook after an acute stroke: urinary incontinence and loss of consciousness compared in 532 patients. *Quarterly Journal of Medicine*, **56**, 601–8.

Wade, D.T. and Hewer, R.L. (1985*b*). Hospital admission for acute stroke: who, for how long, and to what effect? *Journal of Epidemiology and Community Health*, **39**, 347–52.

Wade, D.T. and Hewer, R.L. (1987). Functional abilities after stroke: measurement, natural history and prognosis. *Journal of Neurology, Neurosurgery, and Psychiatry*, **50**, 177–82.

Wade, D.T., Skilbeck, C.E., and Hewer, R.L. (1983*a*). Predicting Barthel ADL score at 6 months after an acute stroke. *Archives of Physical Medicine and Rehabilitation*, **64**, 24–8.

Wade, D.T., Hewer, R.L., Wood, V.A., Skilbeck, C.E., and Ismail, H.M. (1983*b*). The hemiplegic arm after stroke: measurement and recovery. *Journal of Neurology, Neurosurgery, and Psychiatry*, **46**, 521–4.

Wade, D.T., Skilbeck, C.E., Wood, V.A., and Hewer, R.L. (1984*a*). Long-term survival after stroke. *Age and Ageing*, **13**, 76–82.

Wade, D.T., Hewer, R.L., and Wood, V.A. (1984*b*). Stroke: influence of patient's sex and side of weakness on outcome. *Archives of Physical Medicine and Rehabilitation*, **65**, 513–16.

Wade, D.T., Hewer, R.L., and Wood, V.A. (1984*c*). Stroke: the influence of age upon outcome. *Age and Ageing*, **13**, 357–62.

Wade, D.T., Hewer, R.L., Skilbeck, C.E., and David, R.M. (1985*a*). *Stroke: a critical approach to diagnosis, treatment and management*. Chapman and Hall, London.

Wade, D.T., Legh-Smith, J., and Hewer, R.L. (1985*b*). Social activities after stroke: measurement and natural history using the Frenchay Activities Index. *International Rehabilitation Medicine*, **7**, 176–81.

Wade, D.T., Wood, V.A., and Hewer, R.L. (1985*c*). Recovery after stroke—the first 3 months. *Journal of Neurology, Neurosurgery, and Psychiatry*, **48**, 7–13.

Wade, D.T., Hewer, R.L., Skilbeck, C.E., Bainton, D., and Burns-Cox, C. (1985*d*). Controlled trial of a home-care service for acute stroke patients. *Lancet*, **1**, 323–6.

Wade, D.T., Legh-Smith, J., and Hewer, R.L. (1986*a*). Effects of living with and looking after survivors of a stroke. *British Medical Journal*, **293**, 418–20.

Wade, D.T., Parker, V., and Hewer, R.L. (1986*b*). Memory disturbance after stroke: frequency and associated losses. *International Rehabilitation Medicine*, **8**, 60–4.

Wade, J. (1987). Extracranial-intracranial bypass, one; clinical trials, nil. *British Medical Journal*, **295**, 212.

Walker, J.W. (1977). Changing US life style and declining vascular mortality: cause or coincidence. *New England Journal of Medicine*, **297**, 163–5.

Walker, S.R. and Rosser, R.M. (ed.) (1988). *Quality of life: assessment and application*. MTP Press, Lancaster, UK.

Walker, M.G., Shaw, J.W., Thomson, G.J.L. *et al.* (1987). Subcutaneous calcium heparin versus intravenous sodium heparin in treatment of established acute deep vein thrombosis of the legs: a multicentre prospective randomised trial. *British Medical Journal*, **294**, 1189–92.

Warlow, C.P. (1987). Cerebrovascular disease. In *Oxford Textbook of Medicine*, (ed. D.J. Weatherall, J.G.G. Ledingham, and D.A. Warrell), pp. 21.155–21.170. Oxford University Press, Oxford.

Warlow, C.P. and Peto, R. (1987). Extracranial-intracranial bypass, one; clinical trials, nil. *British Medical Journal*, **295**, 211.

Warlow, C.P., Ogsten, D., and Douglas, A.S. (1972). Venous thrombosis following strokes. *Lancet*, **1**, 1305–6.

Weddell, J.M. and Beresford, S.A.A. (1979). *Planning for stroke patients. A four year descriptive study of home and hospital care*. HMSO, London.

Weisberg, L.A. (1988). Diagnostic classification of stroke, especially lacunes. *Stroke*, **19**, 1071–3.

Weisberg, L.A. and Nice, C.N. (1977). Intracranial tumors simulating the presentation of cerebrovascular syndromes. Early detection with cerebral computed tomography (CCT). *American Journal of Medicine*, **63**, 517–24.

Weksler, B. and Lewin, M. (1983). Anticoagulation in cerebral ischaemia. *Stroke*, **14**, 658–63.

Welin, L., Svardsudd, K., Wilhelmsen, L., Larsson, B., and Tibblin, G. (1987). Analysis of risk factors for stroke in a cohort of men born in 1913. *New England Journal of Medicine*, **317**, 521–6.

Wetherley-Mein, G., Pearson, T.C., Burney, P., and Morris, R.W. (1987). Polycythaemia study. A project of the Royal College of Physicians Research Unit. 1. Objectives, background and design. *Journal of Royal College Physicians, London*, **21**, 7–15.

Whisnant, J.P. (1984). The decline of stroke. *Stroke*, **15**, 160–8.

Whisnant, J.P., Fitzgibbons, J.P., Kurland, L.T., and Sayre, G.P. (1971). Natural history of stroke in Rochester, Minnesota, 1945 through 1954. *Stroke*, **2**, 11–22.

Whitehouse, G. (1987). Radiological diagnosis of deep vein thrombosis. *British Medical Journal*, **295**, 801–2.

Whiting, S. and Lincoln, N. (1980). An ADL assessment for stroke patients. *British Journal of Occupational Therapy*, **2**, 44–6.

Wilcox, R.G., Mitchell, J.R.A., and Hampton, J.R. (1986). Treatment of high blood pressure: should clinical practice be based on results of clinical trials? *British Medical Journal*, **293**, 433–7.

Wilkinson, G., Falloon, I., and Sen, B. (1985). Chronic mental disorders in general practice. *British Medical Journal*, **291**, 1302–4.

Williams, J., Wenden, F., and Jenkins, D.G. (1984). Speech therapy for aphasic stroke patients. *Lancet*, **1**, 1413.

Wilson, B. (1982). Success and failure in memory training following a cerebral vascular accident. *Cortex*, **18**, 581–94.

Winslow, C.M., Soloman, D.H., Chassin, H.R. *et al.* (1988). The appropriateness of carotid endarterectomy. *New England Journal of Medicine*, **318**, 721–7.

Wolf, P.A., Dawber, T.R., Thomas, H.E., and Kannel, W.B. (1978). Epidemiological assessment of chronic atrial fibrillation and risk of stroke. The Framingham study. *Neurology*, **28**, 973–7.

Wolf, P.A., D'Agostino, R.B., Kannel, W.B., Bonita, R., and Belanger, A.J. (1988). Cigarette smoking as a risk factor for stroke. The Framingham study. *Journal of the American Medical Association*, **259**, 1025–9.

Wood, P. and Badley, E. (1978). An epidemiological appraisal of disablement. In *Recent advances in community medicine*, (ed. A.E. Bennett). Churchill Livingstone, London.

Wood-Dauphinee, S., Shapiro, S., Bass, E. *et al.* (1984). A randomized trial of team care following stroke. *Stroke*, **15**, 864–71.

WHO (World Health Organization) (1978). Cerebrovascular disease: a clinical and research classification. WHO Offset Series No. 43. WHO, Geneva.

WHO (World Health Organization) (1980). The international classification of impairments, disabilities and handicaps. WHO, Geneva.

WHO/ISH Mild Hypertension Liaison Committee (1982). Trials of the treatment of mild hypertension. An interim analysis. *Lancet*, **1**, 149–56.

Wylie, C.M. (1967). Measuring end results of rehabilitation of patients with stroke. *Public Health Reports*, **82**, 893–8.

Index